Valuation
of Veterinary Practices

Also in the Practice Ownership Series

Buying a Veterinary Practice

Compensation Models for Owners, Associates, and Staff

Starting a Veterinary Practice

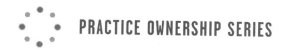

PRACTICE OWNERSHIP SERIES

Valuation
of Veterinary Practices

Understanding the Theory, Process, and Report

2ND
EDITION

AAHA
press

Lorraine Monheiser List, CPA, CVA

American Animal Hospital Association Press
12575 West Bayaud Avenue
Lakewood, Colorado 80228 USA
303/986-2800 or 800/883-6301
press.aahanet.org

ISBN-13: 978-1-58326-145-3

Library of Congress Cataloging-in-Publication Data

Monheiser-List, Lorraine, 1947-
  Valuation of veterinary practices : understanding the theory, process, and report /
Lorraine Monheiser List. — 2nd ed.
    p. ; cm.
  ISBN 978-1-58326-145-3 (pbk. : alk. paper)
  1. Veterinary medicine—Practice—Valuation. 2. Veterinary medicine—Economic aspects. I.
American Animal Hospital Association. II. Title.
  [DNLM: 1. Practice Valuation and Purchase—methods. 2. Hospitals, Animal—economics. 3.
Practice Management—economics. SF 756.4]
  SF756.4.M674 2008
  636.089'0681—dc22
                        2010031009

This information is intended to help you make good management decisions, but it is not a replacement for appropriate financial, legal, or other advice. Neither AAHA nor the author assumes responsibility for or makes representation about the suitability or accuracy of the information contained in this work for any purpose, and makes no warranties, either express or implied, including the warranties of merchantability and fitness for a particular purpose. Neither AAHA nor the author shall be held liable for adverse reactions to or damage resulting from the application of this information or any misstatement or error contained in this work. AAHA and the author shall be held harmless from any and all claims that may arise as a result of any reliance on the information provided.

Book design by Erin Johnson Design

Printed in the United States of America

11 12 13 / 1 2 3 4 5 6 7 8 9 10

Contents

Preface

Whether you are looking at a valuation for the purpose of buying, selling, or merging a practice; obtaining financing for the practice or owner; establishing or maintaining an employee stock ownership plan; or updating your strategic plan, this book will help you reach your goal. You will gain an understanding of what valuation is and how it has evolved within the veterinary profession (Chapter 1). You will be walked through the valuation process step by step to gain greater understanding of valuations and how they are prepared (Chapters 2, 4, and 5), and you will learn what to look for in an appraiser and how to make the best choice for your purpose (Chapter 3). You will be taught how to evaluate a report prepared by an appraiser (Chapter 6), and finally, you will be provided with a case study to help you explore what valuation means in a specific fact pattern and how a valuation might impact you, your practice, or a practice you hope to acquire (Chapter 7).

As you read the chapters, keep in mind that there is no one-size-fits-all approach to valuations. The appraisal process will differ depending on the purpose of the valuation and the underlying facts, as will the finished product. The insight provided in these pages will help you develop an awareness of how an outsider might view your practice, or how you should view a practice that is not yours. It will give you the information you need to build your practice up and increase its value. And it will help ensure that, whether you buy or sell a practice, it will be at the best price.

Finally, please understand that this book is not a "cookbook" approach to valuation. Its goal is not to teach you how to prepare a valuation but to expand your understanding of valuations you will encounter during your years in practice. It is designed to give you insight into the valuation process so that you can ask the right questions—and know how to interpret the answers—when it is time for you to make use of the services of a valuation expert. Keep in mind that, in any individual transaction, you may be talking to the appraiser as a current owner of a practice or as a potential purchaser. Your knowledge of the appraisal process is important in both instances, and you have both a right and an obligation to ask enough questions to understand how the value was determined.

Introduction
The Evolution of Veterinary Practice Valuations

This book is divided into seven major parts:

- A discussion of the evolution of valuations as they relate to veterinary practices
- Steps in the valuation process and the theory behind each
- Tips on how to find an appraiser and how to save time and money if it's your practice being valuated
- Basic valuation theory and methods
- A description of the process used in the valuation of veterinary practices and an in-depth discussion of the components involved
- A discussion of how to analyze an appraisal, even if done for a practice you don't own currently, including ways to judge the reasonableness of the appraiser's methods and conclusions
- A case study to demonstrate one set of facts and the appraiser's determination of value

Because the valuation process is an attempt to estimate the price on which a buyer and a seller would agree, it is never cut-and-dried or reducible to simple formulas. The expectations of buyers and sellers and the value levels themselves will fluctuate with changes in the veterinary profession and in the economy. The veterinary profession is dynamic, and the valuation of veterinary practices must therefore also be dynamic.

Defining the Terms

Adjusted book value: the difference between the practice's total assets (restated to their current value) less its total debts (also adjusted to their current value, if needed).

Adjusted profit: historical net profit as adjusted by the valuator during the valuation process.

Book value: the difference between the practice's total assets (recorded at original cost) and its total debts (as shown on its financial statements).

Capitalization (or cap) rate: a percentage representing risk that is divided into adjusted profits to convert those profits to a value.

Capitalized earnings: adjusted profit divided by a percentage that represents risk, with the result representing value (for example: $1,000 capitalized at 25% = $4,000, or $1,000 ÷ 0.25).

Discount rate: a rate of return used to convert a future sum into its present value.

Discounted earnings: a stream of future earnings, restated to its value today by applying a discount rate (for example: $1,000 per year for 10 years is worth $7,722 at an interest rate of 5%).

Earnings multiple: the reciprocal of the capitalization rate (for example: a 25% cap rate = a multiple of 4).

Goodwill: an intangible asset that represents the difference between total value and the value of the tangible assets included in adjusted book value.

Gross receipts: the total of all the fees or other income the practice earns or collects.

Intangible asset: something of value that has no physical characteristics, such as goodwill or going-concern value.

Net profit (or net income): the practice's gross receipts reduced by the sum of all its expenses.

Return on investment: the dollars an investor can expect to earn from practice ownership, which is separate from compensation for services provided or rent on practice facilities.

Tangible asset: something of value that can be seen, touched, or counted, such as cash, inventory, or equipment.

The emergence of national consolidators—companies whose objective it is to acquire and operate multiple veterinary practices—for example, has brought about significant changes in how veterinary businesses are owned and operated. These buyers have purchasing criteria that are unique to them, and this impacts how a target practice's data may be evaluated. Because the consolidators can afford to buy larger practices, this trend affects the veterinary specialties just as much as it does general practice.

Equally important to the valuation process is the number of lenders now in the veterinary field. Even with tightened credit policies, lenders have discovered that loaning money to veterinarians to acquire existing practices or start new ones is good business. These lenders are willing to loan money on the basis of the practice's expected cash flow, not just on the value of tangible assets (equipment, inventory, real estate, etc.) as collateral. As a result, the number of sales in which the seller finances the buyer has decreased dramatically. In today's market, sellers are more likely to receive cash instead of promissory notes when their practices sell. But sellers cannot set their price arbitrarily, as happened all too frequently in the past. When the seller was also the lender, the buyer had less ability to challenge the asking price. Now an outside lender will do an independent analysis to ensure that a practice's cash flow will be sufficient for the buyer to make the payments on the acquisition loan.

A significant increase in the number of specialty and emergency practices has also had an impact on practice valuations. There is much less similarity between one specialty referral practice and another than there is among general veterinary practices, even though every practice is still unique. Also, the legal, financial, and operating structure of referral practices can be quite complex. Because of their complexity and uniqueness, valuing specialty practices is becoming a niche within veterinary practice valuation and is not for the inexperienced or the fainthearted.

Today, buyers, lenders, and appraisers increasingly emphasize profits and cash flow in determining practice value. While buying a practice generally includes purchasing inventory and equipment, those items by themselves have limited value.

After all, cash, equipment, inventory, and hospital facilities don't generate profits by themselves. Successful veterinary practices, including specialties, hire doctors and staff, develop relationships with referring veterinarians and clients, and devise internal systems to provide quality patient care and client service. It's the combination of all those factors that drives practice value.

While multiples (or fractions) of gross receipts used to be common in determining value, most thoughtful appraisers now use some variation of capitalized or discounted earnings, creating an adjusted book value that includes goodwill and is based on actual practice profits. They know that the profitability of a practice has a major impact on its value, but they also know that actual practice profits may vary significantly from the net income figure on the practice's profit-and-loss statement. True profits can be significantly different because of operating decisions owners make and legitimate tax-planning opportunities they use that serve to reduce income or payroll taxes by lowering reported profits in some or all years.

Changes in the Field

Interest in veterinary practice valuation has increased steadily since the 1970s and 1980s. Several developments coincided to create this interest.

First, there were simply many more practices being bought and sold than there were in earlier decades. In bygone days, veterinarians were more likely to keep their businesses small, preferring to remain as sole owners of their practices. They were inclined to stay put, and there were not as many sales or purchases of practices as we now see. As practitioners who started their practices in the 1940s, 1950s, or 1960s reached or approached retirement age, they became interested in selling their practices at the best possible price, creating a market for valuation services.

Second, as the baby boomers graduated from the veterinary schools and began their careers, there were more practitioners looking for positions, seeking to start new clinics, or searching for practices that could be purchased. The number of practices in existence increased throughout the country.

Third, inflation and rising costs caused veterinarians' fees and the value of their practices to creep up. As a result, the average selling price of practices increased. Therefore, the purchase or sale of a veterinary practice came to represent a major investment with major tax consequences. Obtaining professional assistance in the valuation and tax-planning realm for such a transaction became more necessary and more commonplace.

Fourth, different lenders entered the marketplace who were willing to finance practice startups and acquisitions, which meant that the seller no longer had to also be the lender. However, the new lenders set certain criteria for buyers in order to protect themselves from default, and one of the main considerations was the practice's expected cash flow.

Finally, as larger national corporations entered the pet-care industry, they gave sellers an option that had not previously existed: Instead of selling their practice to another practitioner, they could now sell to a corporation that operated many clinics within a region or around the country. Practice owners needed help in understanding and evaluating these corporate purchase offers. Was the offering price reasonable in light of the seller's other options?

The effect on the valuation of veterinary practices was dramatic. As interest in the subject of valuation itself increased, the way buyer/seller negotiations proceeded underwent some important changes. There was now more analysis based on concrete data to guide the way deals were struck.

Because more practices were changing hands, more practitioners were interested in having an outside opinion of how much their practices were worth. Although there had always been sales and purchases of veterinary practices, the deals had often been quietly negotiated by the parties involved and resulted in long-term promissory notes from buyer to seller. The seller was frequently, though not always, an older and more experienced businessperson who could negotiate a fairly high value, since the buyer typically had few options. The buyer, looking at the other career opportunities available, often picked a locale and then focused primarily on whether he or she thought the monthly payments were "doable." Rules of thumb based on gross fees provided a quick and easy way to set a price.

After the sale, there were several possible outcomes. In the happy scenarios, the buyer made the payments and was able to pay himself or herself a reasonable salary. The new owner might struggle financially in the early years, but the practice still grew, became more profitable, and provided a comfortable life for the owner. In the worst-case scenarios, the buyer faltered. If the price was too high and the cash flow too low for the owner to make the payments, the buyer either had to settle for a less-than-ideal salary or was forced to default on the payments. Sometimes, the buyer would look at the years of payments still to be made and the hard work required to operate and grow a practice, and conclude that a career change was more appealing. In those cases, the seller may have needed to (and sometimes did) take the practice back. However, the practice that was left to take over was often a shadow of the former practice, and the seller was reluctant to go back to it at that stage in life.

This kind of outcome was common enough that both sellers and buyers became more cautious. Instead of basing value on gross fees, they began to look at net income and cash flow. Most veterinarians had limited knowledge of accounting and finance and were ill equipped to view financial information and reach determinations about assets, liabilities, net income, and cash flow. Buyers and sellers sought help from financial experts who could give them more reliable and detailed information. Both needed to know how to determine whether, at a given price for a practice, the buyer would be able to make the payments and succeed as a practice owner.

The trend toward capitalized earnings and more formal valuations grew. That movement grew even faster as the national corporations emerged. By definition, the corporations were never going to have the emotional attachment to any practice that either the seller or an individual buyer might have. Instead they viewed a purchase as a pure business decision: If we invest this many dollars in a target practice, how long will it take to get our money back? How much (or how little) can we pay up front, and can we buy part of the practice with our own company stock, thereby lowering our cash requirements? Can we make adjustments to operations to increase the target's profitability and recoup our money faster? Although the gross amount of client fees was relevant to such buyers, it was estimations of future net profit and cash flow that drove (and still drive) their purchase decisions.

This trend has led to more analysis and more complexity in valuations, but it has also led to better valuations. If a valuation is done properly, it gives both buyer and seller the information they need to feel comfortable about entering into the transaction. And since such arm's-length transactions are the cornerstone of fair market value, it has become vital to buy or sell a practice at a price that is reasonable to both parties.

Constants in a Changing Environment

Though the valuation of veterinary practices is dynamic and complex, some standardization is not only possible but desirable. Indeed, over the past few decades the valuation of veterinary practices has moved toward more standardization rather than less. In past years some valuators followed their own procedures and set their own priorities, frequently independent of established valuation theory. Their underlying belief was that veterinary practices were totally different from other small businesses. If that was ever true, it certainly is no longer the case. The gap between valuation methods for veterinary practices and other kinds of small businesses has narrowed. There will always be some differences in the conclusions reached by different appraisers, since in all valuations there is an element of professional judgment. But many valuation standards are now commonly accepted by valuation experts as well as by lenders, courts, and taxing authorities. What are those constants in veterinary practice appraisals?

- There will never be a quick and dirty rule of thumb for valuing practices, much as everyone would like to have one.

- Practices that are overpriced will take much longer to sell, if they sell at all. More and more, buyers are getting outside advice to ensure that the asking price is reasonable.
- Sellers cannot demand artificially high prices by offering to finance the purchase.
- Buyers who pay too much for a practice face years of stress while they try to operate a struggling practice and repay the money they borrowed to make the purchase.
- Sellers play a key role in transitioning ownership and setting buyers up for success.
- Practice owners have a right to a reasonable return on the dollars invested in a practice, though owners will disagree about what's "reasonable."
- The value of a practice is never a single figure—it is actually a range of reasonable values for that practice at a particular point in time and for a particular purpose.

2

The Valuation Process
What to Expect

Certain concepts hold true in business valuation for all types of businesses, and veterinary practices are no exception. It is a deliberate process characterized by specific steps, exchanges of information, and communication of the results. By knowing these steps, you can help ensure that the valuation process for your practice goes smoothly and increase the likelihood of an accurate assessment that meets your needs.

But valuation of veterinary practices is also unique, with many considerations that do not apply to other types of businesses. In this chapter, you'll get an overview of the valuation process as it applies specifically to veterinary practices.

The Appraisal Process: An Overview

An appraiser must take the following steps to reach a reasonable conclusion as to value.

Step 1. Determine the purpose of the valuation.

Step 2. Determine if equity or assets are being valued.

Step 3. Determine the standard and premise of value.

Step 4. Establish the effective date of the valuation.

Step 5. Gather information.

Step 6. Adjust historical financial information as needed.

Step 7. Establish value using one or more methods.

Step 8. Report the results.

We will take these steps in sequence in the sections that follow to help you navigate the valuation process. In later chapters, you'll learn about each step in more detail.

Your Step-by-Step Guide

Step 1. Determine the Purpose of the Valuation

Why would it matter why the valuation is being requested? Wouldn't the value of the practice be the same regardless of the reason it needs to be done? The answer to the second question is a resounding no, because the purpose of the valuation drives both the determination of what is being valued and the proper analysis and adjustments that must be done.

An appraiser needs to know the purpose of the valuation in order to know the kind and amount of detail required and the format of the finished product. For example, a valuation performed for federal estate or gift tax purposes must reach a precise figure as the correct value of the practice for inclusion in tax returns to be filed with the Internal Revenue Service (IRS) or other taxing authorities. Since a range of values is not acceptable to the IRS, additional detail and research may be required to define this value more precisely. The final report may be much longer (and more expensive) than reports done for other purposes because it must fully disclose all the relevant issues as prescribed by the taxing authorities. On the other hand, if partners in a practice need only to know a general value of the practice for life insurance purposes, then a range of values and a shorter report may suffice.

There are many other reasons for having valuations done, and the process, as well as the finished product, will be different for each (see sidebar on "Reasons for Requesting a Valuation").

At the outset, the valuator will want to determine whether you are asking for a *conclusion of value* or a *calculation of value*. For a conclusion of value, the valuator will consider different approaches and methods and choose what he or she feels is most appropriate in arriving at the practice's value. For a calculation of value, he or she will do a mathematical calculation based on a specific set of assumptions and a particular method or set of methods chosen and/or agreed to by the client and the valuator. In a calculation of value, there will likely be little or no consideration of alternate approaches during the valuation process itself.

For example, the written agreement among owners in a multi-owner practice (the "buy-sell agreement") may specify a formula, a method, an effective date of the valuation, and other terms in connection with a specific situation, such as an owner's retirement. In that case, the valuator will make the calculation as requested, but the number the valuator arrives at may not be the same number he or she would have arrived at if the formula had not existed and the valuator had been free to choose the method and assumptions he or she thought best for the situation.

Step 2. Determine If Equity or Assets Are Being Valued

The appraiser must next determine what kind of interest is being valued: Is it an interest in the practice's assets, or is it an interest in the equity, defined as the difference between its assets and its liabilities? The result of the valuation will be different depending on what is being valued.

For example, if an associate is buying a 20% interest in a practice, he or she is effectively buying an undivided 20% interest in all the practice's assets (cash, equipment, inventory, accounts receivable, and goodwill) and assuming an undivided 20% share of the practice's debts as of the date of the valuation. Therefore, associate buy-ins generally represent the purchase of an equity interest.

Reasons for Requesting a Valuation

All of the following can be reasons for requesting a valuation of a veterinary practice. Your appraiser will perform the valuation with the specific purpose in mind.

- Determining values for estate tax or gift tax
- Buying or selling a practice in its entirety
- Buying or selling a partial interest in a practice
- Strategic planning to evaluate whether current operations are building long-term value
- Obtaining financing for the practice or for an owner
- Establishing or maintaining an employee stock ownership plan
- Granting options to acquire stock in a practice
- Divorcing a spouse or signing a prenuptial agreement
- Determining life insurance or other insurance needs

In the purchase of an entire practice, however, buyers almost always are acquiring the practice's assets, but not assuming any of the practice's debts. Instead, the seller uses the sales proceeds to pay off the practice's obligations to its vendors or other creditors. In that case, the appraiser is determining the value of an interest in the assets, but will not reduce that value by any of the practice's debts unless the buyer specifically agrees to assume that obligation. Therefore, an appraisal of an asset interest will almost always generate a higher value than an appraisal of an equity interest, even for the same practice and at the same point in time, since practices generally do have some debt.

Step 3. Determine the Standard and Premise of Value

Most people are familiar with the term "fair market value" because it is the most common standard of value in home ownership. Fair market value works basically the same way in veterinary practices as it does in residential sales. It is defined as "the price at which property would change hands between a willing buyer and a willing seller when the former is not under any compulsion to buy and the latter is not under any compulsion to sell, both parties having reasonable knowledge of all the relevant facts."

Fair market value assumes a hypothetical buyer from a universe of potential buyers and is therefore not specific to any particular buyer. This is the appropriate standard for valuations prepared for income or estate tax purposes and for some valuations even when no actual sale is contemplated. For example, appraisals being performed for partners in a practice who want to ensure that they have enough life insurance to buy out a deceased owner will likely use a fair market value standard.

However, fair market value is only one of three standards of value that might be used in determining the value of a business, two of which are used frequently in veterinary practice appraisals. (The third relates to shareholder disputes resulting from actions taken or not taken within a company and is generally not relevant here.) Instead of fair market value, a veterinary appraiser might use "investment value," which is based on a specific buyer's investment or strategic objectives, and therefore on situations that might be different from those of a hypothetical buyer.

If, for example, a veterinarian already owned a practice near the one being appraised, she might be willing to pay more for that practice than a hypothetical buyer because her strategy was to combine the two practices into her current facility without incurring a significant increase in fixed costs.

Investment value is also the appropriate standard to use when an associate is buying a noncontrolling interest (less than 50.1%) in an existing practice. In that case, the appraiser cannot make the same assumptions concerning the future operations of the practice as he or she would for a fair market value appraisal. The current owners may already have agreements in place regarding salaries, rent, and other operating details, and all of these prior agreements need to be taken into consideration. Although a buyer of 100% of the practice could make whatever operational changes he or she wanted, an associate buying 10% will have limited control over future decision-making, and the valuation needs to reflect this.

Appraisers use the term "premise of value" to refer to underlying assumptions about the circumstances of the business being valued. For example, in most cases, the valuator is assuming that a veterinary practice will stay in operation and will continue to function as a going concern. Other assumptions might relate to the value as an assemblage of assets not currently being used in a business (and sitting in storage, for example), value in an orderly disposition (generally on an asset-by-asset sale over an extended period of time), or liquidation value in a forced sale.

Step 4. Establish the Effective Date of the Valuation

The effective date of a valuation is more important than the average person might assume. The value of a business changes from day to day, week to week, month to month, and year to year. While a valuation based on a date one week ago is probably still relevant to your decision-making process, a valuation based on a date three years ago is probably not very relevant, or at least of limited relevance, to anything you would be doing today.

Choosing the Effective Date of the Valuation

Choose the effective date carefully if you are hiring a valuator, and assess the reasonableness of the date chosen if you are reviewing an appraisal of a target practice in a purchase or a merger. For practices that are growing rapidly or that have experienced a recent adverse event, such as the loss of a valued associate doctor or the opening of a strong competing practice nearby, the choice of the effective date can be very material.

Consider also that many practices keep their financial records internally, with their CPA making any needed adjustments only at year-end. Using unadjusted financial statements throughout the year can materially distort the practice's financial position in the most recent period, since the accuracy and completeness of internal accounting vary widely among practices. Choosing a valuation date that coincides with the practice's year-end for tax purposes generally results in better financial data.

Practices with a limited history (three years or less) may have experienced losses in the first year or two but then started generating profits at an increasing rate. Choosing a later effective date may well result in a higher practice value. Conversely, valuing a practice as of a date prior to some negative event may result in an artificially high value, especially if the event is likely to have long-term consequences or recur in the future.

But that does not mean that a valuation based on a date three years ago would never be relevant or desirable: Sometimes valuations are done for a particular point in the past for a specific reason—for example, to get an accurate snapshot of the value of the business on the date of an owner's death. The valuation might need to be done at the end of the practice's normal accounting year or at the end of a certain month. Whatever the effective date is, all of the information used for the valuation should be tied to the same point in time. For example, an appraiser should not use a financial statement from December 31 and adjust it by accounts receivable or inventory from September 30.

Step 5. Gather Information

Gathering all the necessary data is frequently the most time-consuming part of a valuation and also the most critical. If the appraiser doesn't have accurate and sufficient data, both about the industry and about the business itself, the results of the valuation can be significantly misleading.

If you are the practice owner, the valuator will tell you what information he or she would like to see, and it's important for the data you provide to be as complete and accurate as possible. As the business owner, your input during this phase is vital. Understand that the more information the valuator has about the practice, the better and more accurate the result will be. Don't hesitate to discuss with the valuator the practice history, unusual events in the past, and nonrecurring expenses from any given year or to provide additional documents to the appraiser that he or she did not specifically request. (See Chapters 4 and 5 for more information about gathering data for your appraiser. Steps 5 through 7 are also discussed in further detail in Chapter 5.)

If you are not the practice owner, see if the valuation report lists the data provided to the appraiser, a standard feature in a normal valuation report. This allows you to determine whether the valuator had a reasonable amount of data about the practice and how it operates. In particular, look for how many years' worth of data were provided and for legal agreements that might impact future operations, such as employment contracts with associates and facility leases.

Step 6. Adjust the Historical Financial Information

During the appraisal process, the appraiser may make many modifications to the company's historical financial and accounting information. This does not mean there was any problem with the company's recordkeeping; it simply reflects the fact that normal practice accounting is sometimes different from the accounting needed for a valuation.

Normal practice accounting uses different rules and serves a purpose different from that of accounting for a valuation. Most practice recordkeeping is done to meet tax or other external requirements. Furthermore, it is done under accounting principles specifying that all transactions be recorded at cost. All items of value (such as a building or equipment) are also reported at cost, whether they have increased or decreased in value since they were purchased.

A business appraiser must make adjustments to the financial statements to develop the information required for valuation purposes. Several of the common adjustments are discussed in the case study that appears in Chapter 7.

Step 7. Establish Value Using One or More Methods

The actual calculation of value is done using one or more established valuation methodologies. These include capitalized earnings approaches, excess earnings approaches, discounted future earnings approaches, and book value or adjusted book value approaches (each will be defined in Chapter 4). The choice of method is critical, and no one method is appropriate for all practices.

Depending on the data available and the unique characteristics of every practice, the appraiser must choose the appropriate method or methods for each valuation he or she performs. Regardless of the choice, the goal is the same: to identify the amount that a hypothetical or specific buyer of a veterinary practice would be willing to pay that would allow him or her to pay all the normal practice expenses, earn a reasonable owner's salary, and generate enough cash flow to repay the debt used to buy the practice. Most owners also expect a return on the initial investment over some number of years, perhaps as few as five, but probably not more than ten.

Step 8. Report the Results

The purpose of the valuation strongly influences the kind of report that should be produced. Reports vary widely in terms of both content and length. You and the valuator should establish at the outset whether you want a complete report, a summary report (which may still be more than thirty pages long), or a one- or two-page letter summarizing the results.

Buyers' Cash Flow Expectations

For valuations done in anticipation of a sale of all or part of a practice, some valuators include a schedule in the report that sets forth the buyer's expected personal cash flow in the first year if the buyer pays the price suggested by the valuation. If you are the potential buyer, it is well worth asking for this kind of schedule to be included. It answers the biggest question that you are likely asking yourself: "If I pay this price, will there be enough money generated by the practice to pay all the expenses, pay me a reasonable salary, provide the funds to make the payments on my loan to buy the practice, and still have some money left over to replace equipment or expand the practice over time?"

Study the following feasibility schedules carefully.

- Did the appraiser assume growth in future practice profits at a fixed rate? Is that rate reasonable?

- Does the schedule suggest that the buyer will use both his or her salary *and* the practice profits to make the loan payments, or just the practice profits? As the buyer, could you afford to use part of your salary to pay off the loan?

- Does the schedule take into account the income and payroll taxes you will owe on your compensation and on the practice profits? Some schedules are prepared on a pretax basis, which ignores the fact that taxes are a fact of life.

- After paying all expenses and servicing the debt, will there still be money available to buy or replace equipment as needed?

Credentialed appraisers may have limitations on the kinds of reports they can issue because of the rules of the governing body for their certifying organization. There are also professional standards regulating the content of the report itself. Be sure that the report you are supposed to receive will have enough detail to meet your needs. Consider asking to see the table of contents or index of a sample report before hiring the appraiser in order to ensure you know what will be included in the report you will receive. If you are the seller, consider what your buyer might want to see in a report.

Remember that the final report will often give a range of values, and that any sale or purchase price that falls within that range is a reasonable value. The high and low ends of the range reflect different underlying assumptions about practice operations, market conditions, and the perceived effect of future events on the practice. An agreement between buyer and seller on those assumptions can narrow the gap between the high and low ends, ultimately converting the range to a single figure. In the absence of such an agreement, an independent appraiser, attempting to arrive at a single number for the value of the practice, usually hits the midpoint of the range.

Still, valuations cannot be reduced to a formula that will consistently yield reasonable results, because no two practices are identical. Not only are there always demographic differences, but there are also innumerable differences in operations, in the mix of services, and in practice philosophies. Some veterinarians exhibit significant business acumen, whereas others "let the business run itself." Over a period of years, these differences will create practices with varying values even if the practice size and location are similar.

3

Choosing a
Practice Appraiser

Now that you understand the basic valuation process, let's take a look at how to choose the right appraiser for your practice. Of course, if you are the buyer, you will most likely have no say in who is hired to prepare the report. However, you can still evaluate whether the choice of appraiser seems appropriate based on the criteria discussed in this chapter.

Getting Started

Just as when choosing an accountant or an attorney, the best place to start when choosing an appraiser for your practice may be with recommendations from colleagues who have had a valuation prepared in the past. Here are useful questions to ask colleagues or professionals making an appraiser recommendation:

- Were they satisfied with the process and with the result?
- What was the process like from the practice's viewpoint?
- Was the valuation completed in a timely manner?
- Was the valuator able to answer questions about the conclusions reached?
- Was the final report well written and understandable by someone not familiar with valuation jargon?

The Interview Process

Even if you receive good recommendations, how do you know whether you are hiring a competent professional? The next step is to schedule an interview. If the appraiser is located in your area, the interview can be face-to-face, but a telephone interview is fine if the appraiser is not nearby. If you are conducting a telephone interview, however, do be sure to speak with the actual appraiser instead of a less experienced employee.

Be sure to interview more than one candidate, and ask questions that will help you differentiate among the contenders, such as those suggested in the sidebar "Questions to Ask When Interviewing an Appraiser." They are designed to help you select the appraiser or appraisal firm that will be the best choice for you and your practice. Brief explanations about each question and guidance for evaluating the answers you receive follow.

Experience

The first few questions you will ask appraisers have to do with their level of experience. The best answers would indicate that the appraiser has done valuations for at least several years and works primarily or exclusively with veterinary practices. Not understanding the veterinary profession or how veterinary practices normally operate would be a major barrier to valuing a practice properly, since there is not a lot of data about veterinary practices available outside the profession.

The second question gives you insight on whether the valuator is familiar with the specific type of practice being valued. By itself, knowing a great deal about companion animal wellness practices is not enough to value a food animal or equine practice properly. It would be better if the appraiser also had experience working with practices like yours.

The third question allows you to evaluate whether practices valued by this person actually sold for a price at, or very near to, the value as determined by the appraiser. Keep in mind that not all appraisals are intended to result in an actual transaction (those performed for strategic planning purposes, for example). Also, not all valuators keep their own databases to track this kind of data. However, asking the question lets you evaluate their experience in light of actual ownership transfers of practices they have valued in the past.

Questions to Ask When Interviewing an Appraiser

1. How many veterinary practice valuations have you done in the past year? In the past five years? How many other types of valuations have you done in the same time periods?

2. Have you valued practices similar to the one currently under consideration in the past? (For example, practices with specialties in companion animals, equine medicine, emergency medicine, exotic animals.)

3. Have any of the practices that you have valued been exposed to the market and sold? If so, how many, and did your value hold up?

4. Who will actually be doing the work on this valuation?

5. What training have you had in business valuation? Who sponsored the class(es) you took? When did you take the class (or classes)?

6. Have you spoken at national veterinary continuing education meetings or taught classes on valuations?

7. Are you a member of VetPartners™?

8. What credentials, if any, do you hold in business valuation? How long have you held these credentials and what requirements do you have for continuing education?

9. Will you make an on-site visit to the practice?

10. Can you provide me with the table of contents or index from a report you prepared that would be similar to the one you would give me?

11. Once you have all the data, how long does it generally take to complete the valuation?

12. What is the approximate cost of the valuation we are discussing?

The fourth question deals with who will actually be doing the work for the appraisal. If the person you are interviewing has less experienced staff or assistants who will be involved in the valuation process, make sure that all their work will be thoroughly reviewed. Using lower-level staff can help control the cost of an appraisal. But to get the experience and expertise you think you are hiring, the person at the top should review, sign, and take full responsibility for the project.

Education

The fifth question relates to the appraiser's level of formal training. Ideally, the appraiser will have taken a series of business valuation courses, not just a single class or two. The sponsor of the classes may have been a valuation-specific continuing education provider; an accounting, legal, or professional organization; or even the company the appraiser works for. The important thing is that the appraiser received in-depth training and has stayed abreast of changes in the field. The knowledge should be current and fresh.

The sixth question is a way of determining if this person has the expertise and communication skills to be asked to speak periodically on valuation issues at national meetings. Speakers on technical topics like valuation must understand their material thoroughly to be able to explain it to audiences who are not well versed in the topic. Ideally, those same communication skills will be used to prepare the valuation report.

The seventh question asks if the valuator is a member of VetPartners™, a national professional association of veterinary consultants and advisers, or of a similar organization. The Veterinary Valuation Resource Council, a part of VetPartners, consists of practice appraisers and brokers who deal with valuation issues on a regular basis and seek to improve the quality of valuations in the profession. Membership in VetPartners and in the council indicates a commitment to quality. (For more information, see www.vetpartners.org.)

Credentials

The eighth question asks whether the valuator has made the effort to be credentialed in business valuation. While a valuation credential is not an essential requirement, there are several organizations that provide specific training in valuation theory and practice. When the valuator holds one of these credentials, it gives you the assurance that he or she has met certain standards. It tells you that the valuator successfully completed a required course of study, passed the testing requirements of that organization, and is committed to ongoing continuing education in valuation theory and practice.

Common credentials are listed in the sidebar "Business Valuation Accreditation."

On-Site Visits

Answers to the ninth question, about on-site visits, depend a lot on proximity. Most appraisers will say they need not visit the practice in person, unless they are geographically close and can see the practice easily as part of the data-gathering process. In most cases, a visit to the premises is a lot like kicking the tires on a used car. It makes you feel as if you were doing something useful but does not provide much information. A better approach is for you to create a video tour of the hospital to send the appraiser, which can be very informative. Walk slowly through the rooms with your video camera and narrate as you go. Point out the same things you would highlight if the appraiser were by your side.

Report-Writing Competence

You will likely not be able to see an entire sample report, because the appraisal is subject to privacy rules. All information given to a valuator is confidential, as is

Business Valuation Accreditation

An appraiser might have one of the following accreditations or certifications:

- ABV (Accredited in Business Valuation, by the American Institute of Certified Public Accountants)
- AIBA (Accredited with the Institute of Business Appraisers)
- AM (Accredited Member of the American Society of Appraisers)
- ASA (Accredited Senior Appraiser of the American Society of Appraisers)
- AVA (Accredited Valuation Analyst of the National Association of Certified Valuation Analysts)
- CBA (Certified Business Appraiser of the Institute of Business Appraisers)
- CVA (Certified Valuation Analyst by the National Association of Certified Valuation Analysts)

the resulting report. It is worth asking the tenth question to get a sample table of contents or index, however, because these pieces will give you some idea of how complete your own report would be if you hired this appraiser. The table of contents or the index will allow you to evaluate whether the report would give you (or other readers of the report) a sufficient level of detail.

Estimated Time Frame

The answers to the eleventh question, regarding how long it will take to receive a report, will vary widely. Remember that it's your job to provide the data and answer questions in a timely manner. Expect the process to take at least two months, once the appraiser has the data from the original request. However, an answer indicating a longer time frame does not necessarily mean you should not use this appraiser. Some excellent valuation experts are very busy and may be backlogged for several weeks or months. However, you will want to make sure the approximate date or time frame meets your needs.

Keep in mind that it takes time to do a complete and thorough analysis and prepare the final report. Remember, too, that it's your job to provide the data and answer questions in a timely manner.

Cost

As with most things in life, you get what you pay for, and quality valuations don't come cheap. Question 12 allows you to get an idea of what this appraiser normally charges. Keep in mind that whether the project is a conclusion or calculation of value (see Chapter 2), as well as the kind of report you are requesting, will have an impact on its cost.

Beyond finding out how much the valuation will cost, this is your chance to inquire about how much of the cost, if any, should be paid at the time you hire the appraiser and what the payment terms will be during the process and up to the conclusion of the project.

As you evaluate the answers you receive to all twelve questions, also consider whether the appraiser established good rapport, responded in a timely way to your inquiry, and provided appropriate follow-up with an engagement letter and the list of information needed. Intangible factors such as these can help you identify a professional who will fit well with your communication style. These answers can also be the deciding factor if you have eliminated some of the candidates and are having trouble deciding among the ones who remain.

Necessary Data

Once you have chosen an appraiser, the next part of the process is to begin accumulating the data he or she asks to see. A fair amount of this is financial data (see sidebar "Gathering Data for Your Appraiser").

A valuator understands that it takes time to locate the requested information, but make sure you know when he or she is expecting to receive it, and let the valuator know if there will be any delay. Though it may seem easier for you to send the data piecemeal, as it often comes from different sources, from the standpoint of efficiency it is helpful to send it in no more than two or three batches. It takes time (and costs you money) if the valuator must pick up and put down your file numerous times as the information comes in.

If your situation warrants submitting data in parts, prioritize sending the tax returns and financial statements. These items generally give the valuator enough information to get started, and he or she can begin to make a list of follow-up questions. When you do not have, or are unable to get, the requested items, let the valuator know as soon as possible. He or she may be able to suggest alternate ways for you to provide the necessary information.

Remember that you know more about your practice than anyone else. So if you believe that something not on the list of requested materials would be helpful to the valuator, don't hesitate to include it or ask if it would be helpful. If there

Gathering Data for Your Appraiser

Your appraiser will ask you to gather the data he or she will need to compile your report. That information will likely include most, if not all, of the following:

- Income tax returns
- Year-end financial statements
- Production reports
- Accounts receivable balances
- Inventory on hand
- Equipment lists
- Employment contracts with owners and associates
- Owners' (buy-sell) agreements
- Equipment and facility leases
- Insurance policies
- Information about fee structure, client history, and referring practices, if applicable
- Information about non-doctor employees, their job responsibilities, and their rates of pay
- Information about prior changes in practice ownership
- Information about unusual events in prior years (such as relocations, nonrecurring legal expense, and major facility repairs)
- Information about past and current marketing strategies
- Information about retirement plans and contributions for owners and employees
- Information about competitors

Since the information requested varies somewhat from appraiser to appraiser, other data will likely be needed, both at the outset and during the valuation process, so don't be surprised if the list provided here is incomplete. (For more information on gathering data, see Chapter 5.)

Tips for Efficient Delivery of Data to Your Appraiser

Tip 1. Consider asking your tax preparer to send electronic copies of your complete tax returns directly to the valuator, since many tax programs now make that easy. There's no reason for you or someone on your staff to stand at the copy machine for hours if there's an easier way.

Tip 2. You may find that scanning employment contracts and leases is more efficient for you and gives the appraiser the ability to review the entire document. Even though some of these documents are lengthy, don't try to guess which pages the appraiser should receive, since incomplete documents often result in follow-up questions and requests to send the entire document anyway.

Tip 3. If there are appendices to your lease, or if there were amendments to employment contracts or owners' agreements, be sure to include those as well to avoid follow-up requests.

Tip 4. If you photocopy documents, ask the appraiser before you copy them double-sided. Although it saves paper to copy data onto both sides, it can be a nightmare to try to read those documents when they are fastened down in a file.

Tip 5. If you photocopy documents, check the copies to be sure each page is readable and the copies are complete. Sheet feeders on copy machines are notorious for reproducing only part of the data on a page because the original didn't feed through the machine completely.

have been unusual events or transactions over the past few years, be sure that information is provided to the appraiser. Providing complete and accurate data is your responsibility, and doing so will ensure an accurate and comprehensive finished product.

Finally, ask questions during the appraisal process. You are relying on the appraiser's knowledge of valuation theory, his or her experience with other practices, and his or her understanding of your practice. You should view the process as a learning tool. By asking questions about what the appraiser does and why it is important, you will gain a great deal of insight into significant characteristics of other veterinary practices and their effect on practice value.

4

Communicating Effectively about Appraisals

A complete discussion of valuation theory and methods is certainly beyond the scope of this book, as is the goal to teach you how to do valuations. If you can acquire a good understanding of the basic concepts in valuation, however, you will be able to communicate more effectively with an appraiser, whether you are the practice owner or the user of a valuation report. You will have a better grasp of what he or she is trying to accomplish and why, and you will be ready to aid him or her in ways that help produce a report that is as accurate as possible. You will also be more comfortable challenging assumptions or adjustments because you understand the implications and consequences of each. Some of the main concepts of valuation theory are explained here with these purposes in mind; they also reflect some of the work done in step 7 of the process outlined in Chapter 1.

Whether to Use Rules of Thumb

Most businesspeople know a few things about appraisals. They have heard or read about them enough to have bits and pieces of knowledge. And one thing that most have heard is that sometimes in appraisals, a simple rule of thumb can be used to value a business such as a veterinary practice. As a result, probably the most frequently asked question that veterinarians pose to an appraiser is whether a rule of thumb will work to value the practice.

For many years, professional practices, including veterinary clinics, traded on a multiple or fraction of annual gross revenue. The figure used could be either the most recent year's sales or an average of the past few years. Although no one knows the origin of this rule of thumb, veterinary practices were often assumed to be worth one times gross, and variations of that myth persist today. Based on this rule of thumb, a clinic grossing $1 million a year would be worth around $1 million. Real estate, if owned by the practice or practice owner, would be valued separately.

At first blush, using a rule of thumb like this may seem like a good idea. If it worked, it would be an easy way to come up with a figure, and the determination could be made very quickly and at greatly reduced expense. However, the values arrived at in this way are almost never valid, and it would likely be only a coincidence if a rule of thumb yielded the same result as a professional appraisal where all the valuation criteria have been considered.

With just a little digging, it is easy to see why it can be dangerous to rely on a figure arrived at by rule of thumb. Say Practice 1 grosses $1 million but nets $250,000 after all expenses (including the owner's salary), and Practice 2 grosses the same $1 million but nets only $50,000 after paying the owner's salary. Obviously, Practice 1 is worth more than Practice 2, even though the rule of thumb would say they are worth the same amount. Furthermore, what if a significant portion of the $1 million in fees was generated by an associate who just left to work at another clinic nearby? Would your opinion of value change?

Finally, not all practices are marketable. Practices in undesirable areas or ones that can't afford to pay the owner a reasonable salary often don't sell at all. Unless the practice has significant unrealized potential, a buyer will not be willing to acquire that practice at a price higher than the liquidated value of the assets, if at all. The buyer's risk might be lower if he or she started a practice from scratch or shopped for a better practice elsewhere.

Market-Based Methods

A market-based method of valuation would look at similar veterinary practices that were recently sold, find out how much they sold for, and base value on this comparative data. This is how real estate agents determine the asking price for a home. They simply look at similar homes in the area and find out how much purchasers are willing to pay. The number they arrive at by making comparisons among the homes is considered to be fair market value.

In a perfect world, the same thing would work for veterinary practices. We would have a database that tracked the unique characteristics of individual veterinary practices, including selected financial data, along with the actual price each sold for in the open market. Then we could simply match a given practice's data with those of similar practices in the database, and we would have a good approximation of its value.

However, there are no databases in existence with sufficient data on veterinary practices, because the vast majority of practices are privately owned. The sellers and purchasers do not routinely share this kind of information with outside sources. VetPartners is in the process of collecting data on actual practice ownership transitions with the consent of the parties involved. The resulting database will not identify practices by name or location, although it will capture information about the geographic region and certain other data. However, until we have a robust and reliable source of data on veterinary practice ownership transitions like this database, appraisers must use other methods to determine practice value.

Asset-Based Methods

In an asset-based valuation, the appraiser would determine a value for each asset in the practice and then add up the individual values. The resulting figure would represent the total value of the practice. To some extent, this is the logic behind the methods discussed below. However, although asset-based methods may work for some other types of businesses, a pure asset-based approach does not work well for businesses—like veterinary practices—in which the single most valuable asset, goodwill, is an intangible that is generally not even listed on the practice's financial statements.

To shortcut the procedure of valuing each asset in a practice, some people use book value for each item (see the sidebar "Defining the Terms"). Book value might be a fair approximation of the value of a tangible asset (such as a piece of equipment or the items in inventory), but it would be mere coincidence if the book value figure represented the true value of the asset in question.

Adjusted book value comes closer to the true value, and for businesses that are very asset intensive (manufacturing companies, for example), adjusted book value may be a reasonable methodology. A veterinary practice, however, is more than the sum of its tangible assets. Equipment and inventory are valuable, of course, but it is the professional expertise of the doctors and staff and other intangibles, such as goodwill, that make for a successful animal hospital. These intangible assets also need to be quantified as part of the total practice value.

In the absence of a separate appraisal of the practice's equipment and furniture by a qualified personal property appraiser, the value of those assets can only be approximated. In addition, asset-based values don't necessarily reflect how often or how efficiently an asset is used in producing revenue or profit. Giving full value to

Defining the Terms

Book value is an accounting term that represents the original cost of an asset or assets, reduced by an accounting calculation of depreciation that may or may not represent true economic "wear and tear." The practice's overall book value may be further reduced by any outstanding debt.

Adjusted book value adjusts the statements from historical cost to replacement cost of each asset in its current condition. In other words, it does not contemplate restating every asset to the replacement cost of a new one, but rather to the value of the existing asset in its existing condition. This approximates fair market value for that asset.

Liquidation value is what the equipment, inventory, and receivables could be sold for if the practice were being shut down. Liquidation value is generally quite low.

ultrasound equipment that no one in the practice knows how to use, or uses very rarely, may cause the valuator to overvalue the practice's assets. Buyers of practices are buying the profit, or benefit stream, the practice can generate by using its equipment, inventory, and staff, not buying just the assets themselves.

Liquidation value, which assumes a practice is going out of business, puts a zero value on the intangibles. While some businesses may be "worth more dead than alive," they are in the minority. Liquidation value is used only when the value of the assembled assets on liquidation is greater than the earnings that can be generated from those assets. This almost never happens in professional practices unless the only doctor is unable to practice. Therefore, for purposes of determining the value of an ongoing practice, this method does not produce reasonable results.

These asset-based methods may come into play at some point during your appraisal. Certainly, your appraiser will want to see equipment and inventory lists and will ask for information about these items. But your appraiser must use another method, or a combination of methods, to estimate the true value of the practice as a whole.

Income-Based Methods

Because the necessary data for market-based methods aren't available, and because the largest asset in a veterinary practice is usually

Defining the Terms

EBITDA stands for Earnings Before Interest, Taxes, Depreciation, and Amortization, and it is becoming more and more common in discussions of profitability. For most purposes, it basically means "profits." In the valuation context, it can mean adjusted profits as defined in Chapter 1, but before subtracting interest, taxes, depreciation, and amortization. It's not just a complicated way of saying "profits," though, because it is also a complete technical definition of what those "profits" truly are: revenues minus expenses, but before subtracting interest, taxes, and depreciation and amortization figures.

goodwill, an intangible, which makes asset-based methods awkward, most valuators use one of the income-based methods to determine practice value. Here, we will look at three income-based approaches: capitalized earnings methods, the excess earnings method, and the discounted cash flow (or discounted earnings) method.

Capitalized Earnings Methods

Capitalized earnings methods are an assortment of approaches with a common thread: They all make use of (1) a net earnings figure divided by (2) a percentage representing risk and a reasonable rate of return.

The variations come from deciding what earnings figure to use (average, weighted, most recent year, or projected, for example) and what capitalization rate, or expected rate of return, to use. If developed thoughtfully, the earnings figure represents the appraiser's best guess as to what the next year's earnings for the practice will be. The figure will probably be based primarily on historical earnings, with adjustments only for known and quantifiable differences (as opposed to wishful thinking!). In developing the capitalization rate, the appraiser will take several factors into account, including market interest rates, industry risk, the general risk inherent in small businesses, the risk related to the particular business that is the subject of the valuation, and a buyer's expected rate of return.

These methods have support in the marketplace but can skew the results in favor of businesses with low capital investments. In other words, if only cash flow, or earnings, affect the calculation, then a practice with extensive diagnostic or treatment equipment will seem to be worth less than it truly is. The purchase of the equipment reduces the practice's cash flow, which can yield an artificially low figure for the practice's value, particularly if the practice doesn't use that equipment effectively to generate revenue. The practice will get equal treatment to a practice without the same equipment costs only if its earnings are proportionately higher. New equipment does not always translate into higher earnings, especially in the short run. If a practice does have a large investment in tangible assets with low earnings, then an approach other than the income approach may be more appropriate (adjusted book value approach, for example).

Excess Earnings Method

For years, the excess earnings method was the most common method used in valuations of veterinary practices. It was also widely used, and sometimes misused, by the Internal Revenue Service and taxpayers in valuations for gift and estate tax purposes. This method does take goodwill and other intangible assets into account, but, as with any method of valuation, must be used with caution. Some appraisers use the method as an asset-based approach, because it attempts to value different classes of assets, including goodwill.

In general, here is how the excess earnings method works. First, the appraiser determines a value for the net tangible assets of the practice (inventory, equipment, etc.). Next, he or she determines a reasonable rate of return from those tangible assets and multiplies that rate by the value of the net tangible

Defining the Terms

Capitalize means to divide an annual earnings figure by a percentage that represents the risk of achieving those earnings.

Capitalization (or cap) rate is the percentage that represents risk and a buyer's expected return on investment. The annual earnings divided by the capitalization rate represents the value of the investment.

Discount is a method to restate future earnings in today's dollars by applying a factor that reduces them and is based on expected rates of return.

Discounted cash flow is future cash flow brought back to today's dollars by applying a discount as defined above.

Discounted earnings is future earnings brought back to today's dollars by applying a discount as defined above.

Excess earnings is the difference between total adjusted profit and an estimated return on tangible assets.

Keep in mind that we **capitalize** historical earnings and **discount** future earnings.

assets. The result of this calculation is assumed to represent the portion of the net earnings that can be attributed to tangible assets; any earnings above that amount are assumed to be due to goodwill and other intangible assets. To calculate that excess, the appraiser subtracts the figure arrived at above from total net earnings. The difference is then capitalized by dividing these "excess earnings" by a capitalization rate. The practice value is then the sum of the value of the tangible assets and the figure representing capitalized excess earnings, or goodwill.

After establishing this method, the IRS went on record to attack it as not being responsive to changes in the marketplace. Indeed, if the rates of return on tangible and intangible assets that were set forth by the IRS in Revenue Ruling 68-609 are not updated for changes in the economy and in the industry being valued, then the results are meaningless. However, all appraisal methods require judgment on the part of the appraiser, and that may not be the greatest risk in using the excess earnings method.

There are several potential pitfalls inherent in the excess earnings method. First, unless a knowledgeable personal property appraiser is hired to place a true current value on the furniture and equipment, the value of the tangible assets is only an estimate. Most practice owners are not willing to hire an additional appraiser because of the cost of doing so. Therefore, practice appraisers are often forced to put a value on each piece of equipment based only on an estimate of its cost and its age.

When this is added to the fact that many practices don't have a complete, accurate, and detailed listing of their furniture and equipment showing original cost and acquisition date, the resulting estimate becomes little more than a guess. Since the value of these tangible assets is key to dividing up the practice profits into a return on tangibles and the excess earnings on intangibles, the appraiser needs to be careful here. The final result is materially affected if the equipment is not valued properly.

Second, there is no reliable source for finding the expected rate of return on tangible assets. If you purchase ultrasound or digital radiography equipment, what is your expected earnings stream from that equipment? Unfortunately, many practices buy expensive equipment without estimating how much profit, if any, that equipment will generate and over what period of time. Instead, they are focused only on the need to practice quality medicine and take advantage of the latest technology.

As suggested earlier, some practices fail to use their equipment to its revenue-generating potential, in which case the calculated return on tangible assets will be too high and the excess earnings (and resulting goodwill value) too low. Unfortunately, these factors won't simply cancel each other out. Instead, the inaccuracies can lead to valuation results that are not reasonable. This is one area where good communication between the practice owner and the appraiser is essential. Without input from you or someone else at the practice who knows the purpose of the equipment and its value to the practice, a practice valuator can find it extremely difficult to assess how well each piece of equipment is being used.

Discounted Cash Flow (or Discounted Earnings)

This method, sometimes known as discounted future earnings, is based on the theory that a business is worth the present value of the future stream of cash it will generate for the owner(s). Stated differently, the value of a business is the dollar amount today that, if invested at an expected market rate, will generate the same cash as the expected earnings from the business.

To make the actual calculation, the valuator uses projected income and expenses for the next few years, then discounts them—or brings them back to current value—by applying a specific discount rate determined for that practice. Like capitalization rates, discount rates are a reflection of risk. But they differ from capitalization rates because they include an estimate of annual growth. Therefore, the discount rate minus the expected growth rate equals the capitalization rate.

But the method also recognizes that practices don't have an unlimited life. Therefore, there is a second calculation to determine the present worth of a "terminal value" at the end of the forecasted period, which approximates the value inherent in those remaining years.

This methodology is not often seen in the valuation of small businesses and professional practices, but it is very common in other kinds of businesses. Conceptually, it is an excellent method, but it is reliable only when the expected earnings of a business can be estimated with some degree of certainty and an appropriate discount rate can be determined. Budgets with detailed projections are rare in veterinary practices. If it were possible to compare several years of projections done by the practice with the actual results from each of those years, the appraiser could place more reliance on future revenue and expense estimates. Also, there are intangibles that will impact future operating results, including the professional reputation and experience of the doctor(s), which are not easily quantified.

For these reasons, other valuation methodologies are more commonly used for veterinary practice valuations. But there are two notable situations where this method may be the best choice.

- *A newer practice with very little operating history*: In this case, projections may be the only way to approximate profits that will be available to the owner. With little or no financial history, one cannot use historical data as the basis of the valuation; the appraiser may have to use projections of future revenue and expenses.

- *A practice with significant anticipated changes in either revenue or expenses*: For example, if the practice is adding a new line of services that will be generated by doctors and staff who are just joining the practice, there are no historical data about the new service. Similarly, a new facility will likely increase both revenue and expenses (though it is important to project whether expenses or income will increase more).

Although the margin for error in a valuation based on future profits is higher because of the risk of overly optimistic estimates, it is unreasonable to expect a buyer to purchase a practice based on historical earnings when the underlying facts are about to change. Be careful to review the assumptions underlying these estimates for reasonableness, since they will have significant impact on the resulting value. Be particularly attentive to projections that include significant growth in revenue without related increases in expenses. For example, if a practice will produce twice as much revenue five years from now, are doctor and staff wages projected to increase to pay the people who are doing that new work? Are there enough exam rooms to produce twice as much revenue, or will the practice need to remodel or relocate?

Other Methods

The above list is certainly not all-inclusive. Other methods of business valuation exist in the marketplace. Some are combinations of the above or are based on formulas agreed to in advance by co-owners in a practice or by specific buyers and sellers. The ones listed above, however, are the ones your appraiser will be most likely to draw from when determining the value of the veterinary practice. Now that you are familiar with the choices and some of the advantages and disadvantages of each, you will be better able to discuss your practice and its unique circumstances with your appraiser. Similarly, if you are the buyer or considering a merger with this practice, plan on asking the seller or the appraiser your questions in light of the explanations above.

Choosing a Valuation Method

Your appraiser will choose a valuation method based on the information you supply and your answers to his or her questions about your practice. Every practice is unique. What's important to understand is that no one method fits all practices, and no standard formula or rule of thumb allows anyone to shortcut the valuation process. Several of the methods described above will produce a reasonable valuation, so long as accurate data are provided, the underlying analysis is thorough, reasonable assumptions are made, and the method or methods selected are properly applied.

If a written agreement among a practice's owners specifies that a particular valuation method or approach must be used in a given situation, then the valuator will not use or consider other methods unless he or she believes the result would be inappropriate or unrealistic. If the valuator feels the approach specified would yield an inaccurate result, he or she will consult with the parties to discuss making a change to the agreement, if possible.

As mentioned earlier, if the appraiser is preparing a valuation based on the language specified in a legal document, he or she is making a *calculation of value*, whereas if he or she is free to choose the most appropriate methods from all the possible options, this is a *conclusion of value*. If the attorney who drafted the agreement was not knowledgeable about valuation theory or was not advised by an appraiser, the method specified for a calculation of value may not be appropriate and may not result in a reasonable estimate of practice value. When it comes to appraisals, a little knowledge can be a dangerous thing. Even if the agreement was drawn up with the advice of an appraiser, if the appraiser was not familiar with veterinary practices in particular, there could be problems.

Agreements that were drawn up many years ago may also present some problems. The specified method may have seemed appropriate at the time the agreement was drawn up, but if the circumstances of the practice have changed, that method could now be a poor choice. In addition, valuation approaches and methodologies evolve over time, and a methodology that was considered reliable in the past may now be considered questionable. Even good formulas need to be updated periodically.

Sometimes appraisers compute the value using different methods and then average them in some way to come up with a final conclusion of value. While that approach is common in real estate appraisals, it is much less common in business valuations. Because each method requires different types of data and different calculations, most valuators prefer to collect basic information about the practice and then select the most appropriate method based on their judgment and experience, preparing the actual valuation and the report using only one method.

There does not seem to be much support for applying several methods, since the tendency when that is done is to modify the underlying assumptions to get similar results. Generally the facts in a particular situation suggest to an experienced valuator the most appropriate method to use. Also, doing multiple cal-culations takes more time and may increase the cost of the valuation while not improving the result.

It is not surprising that there are possible pitfalls in each of the methods discussed above. The case study that appears in Chapter 7 demonstrates all three methods and suggests potential problem areas in each.

5

The Valuation Process In-Depth
A Guide for Buyers and Sellers

Every valuation follows or should follow a fairly specific process. Valuation is based upon real information and analysis, not speculation and wishful thinking. The final number or range of numbers will have to be justified, both to the person hiring the valuator and to subsequent readers of the valuation report. The appraiser follows a prescribed process, and the numbers are arrived at methodically. They should be easy to present, to explain, and, if necessary, to defend.

However, the final report will only be as accurate as the information the appraiser had to work with. Supplying that information will be up to the practice owner. This chapter will look in depth at the data-gathering stage of the valuation process, step 5 in the eight-step process outlined in Chapter 2. It will also explain additional factors your appraiser will be considering as he or she completes the analysis of the data for steps 6 and 7. Chapter 6 will look in more detail at the last step, the final report itself. For purposes of this discussion, we'll assume that you are the owner of the practice and that you are hiring the appraiser, though it is just as important that a potential buyer of the practice, or any other user of a valuation report, also understands the normal appraisal process.

The Engagement Letter

Steps 1 through 4 of the valuation process, from determining its purpose to establishing the effective date (see Chapter 2), are done very early, generally during the initial interview. Once you select and hire an appraiser, you will be asked to sign an engagement letter setting forth the work to be done.

The engagement letter should reflect the decisions you and the valuator reached concerning steps 1 through 4 in your initial discussions. Controversies concerning valuations often can be traced back to misunderstandings or lack of agreement about what was being valued, the purpose of the valuation, and the appropriate valuation date. Detailed engagement letters are designed to avoid these misunderstandings. So don't just sign it; read it carefully to make sure it reflects your circumstances and expectations.

Gathering Data for the Appraiser

Once you've signed the engagement letter, the appraiser will ask you to supply data. This is step 5, and it will be the most time-consuming part of the process for you. After that step is completed and all the necessary information is in the appraiser's hands, it will be up to him or her to complete the financial analysis and produce the report, though you likely will be asked for clarification of certain items and may also need to provide additional documents or background.

During the data-gathering stage, think outside the box. Your appraiser will request specific pieces of information, but there may be other facts or sets of data pertinent to the practice value that he or she would not think to ask for. This is your opportunity to inform the appraiser as to what you believe makes your practice unique and what might, therefore, cause it to command a higher (or lower) price.

If, for example, you have a specialty that is particularly lucrative but that is combined with other fees on your books, you should point this out to the appraiser. Similarly, if you have developed a new procedure, added a new service, or created a new product that is or appears to be marketable, the appraiser should be made aware of this fact. On the other hand, if revenue was down the prior year because of circumstances beyond your control (for example, a key associate was out for three months with a new baby), you should point this out, too. Otherwise, the appraiser may spend a lot of time looking for clues to determine why revenues fell and wonder if the decrease is a sign of the direction revenues will take in the future.

No matter what it is, if there is a factor that you believe may be relevant, discuss it with the appraiser. Don't assume that he or she will know to ask the question. It is your job to present information about your practice. Any major change up or down, in either assets or income, needs attention, as do changes in financial trends.

As for the information that the appraiser requests, be sure to supply it in as timely a way as possible (see Chapters 2 and 3 for more tips on gathering data). Most appraisers will ask for at least three years of financial statements and income tax returns. Some prefer to receive statements covering a five-year period to facilitate better trend analysis. Copies of buy-sell agreements, partnership agreements, employment contracts, lease agreements, and documents concerning previous purchases or sales of all or a part of the practice should be provided to the appraiser. Keep in mind that more recent events have a greater impact than older ones, so pay more attention to these. Even though you are being asked for information from a three-year or five-year period, be sure to think carefully about what the appraiser might need to know about the past year or two.

Detailed information concerning the practice's fee structure and client history is also important, as it can reveal stability, growth, and other data necessary to determine the degree of risk inherent in the practice. If most of your clients have been with the practice for a number of years, the chances of retaining them for several years into the future are good. On the other hand, if you practice in an area where you have high client turnover—near a military base, for example—you will need to add new clients each year just to keep the practice revenue constant.

If yours is a specialty or referral practice, the appraiser will want to know more about your referring veterinarians and the marketing you are doing to grow your practice. Do most of your referrals come from just a handful of veterinarians, or do you receive referrals from many of the local practices? Do you market your emergency practice to the general public, or are you a referral-only practice? How, and how often, do you keep the referring veterinarian informed about the animal's progress while it is in your care? Which services are your competitors also providing in the specialty or specialties you offer? The answers to these questions provide insight into the likelihood of a continuing revenue stream, since you likely do not have the same repeat clientele that a wellness practice would.

Balance sheets and income statements reveal the financial history of the practice. On the balance sheet, the cash position of the company and its receivables provide insight into the cash-management policies of the business. Liabilities indicate the existing commitments against future cash flow and may indicate stability or instability. A comparison of balance sheets over a multiyear period can reveal the history of the business and, more importantly, can indicate trends for potential growth in income, expenses, or both. Practices that are strapped for cash or have failed to upgrade and maintain equipment suggest issues that a buyer would have to resolve.

Income statements are extremely important for businesses that sell services, and the more detailed the service income categories are, the better the appraiser can determine which areas of the practice are contributing to the bottom line. Frequently the practice management software produces more information on service breakdowns than the hospital's accounting records, which is why the valuator will ask for detail from that software as well. (See sidebar "Other Necessary Items" for more information about what your appraiser will need.)

The Appraiser's Analysis

Step 6, adjusting the historical financial statements of the business, will be done by the appraiser. Even though you won't be directly involved, it is important for you to know, in general, what the appraiser will be considering during this stage. If you have information about the practice that may affect any aspect of the analysis, don't hesitate to bring it up.

Different business valuation experts go through different processes during this step, but the overall objective is the same. At best, historical financial statements record only what happened; they do not record what will happen next year or three years from now. An appraiser can evaluate a practice's financial history, but he

Other Necessary Items

In addition to the information listed elsewhere in this chapter, your appraiser will want to see the following items:

- Production by doctor and salary history by doctor for the same periods as the financial statements
- Copies of employment contracts for owners and associates
- A copy of your current fee schedule (to allow for comparisons of your charges with others' fees for the same or similar services)
- A copy of the title page from life insurance policies for each of the owners, as well as information on the annual premiums and whether those are paid by the practice or the individual owners
- A copy of your current lease of the clinic facilities, regardless of whether you are renting from an unrelated party or from one or more of the doctors

- Additional information about the duties, hours worked, and salaries of spouses or other family members on the hospital's payroll
- Information about retirement plans for owners and employees, such as 401(k) and SIMPLE plans
- Any information about "hidden" assets that the practice owns (such as equipment or supplies that have been expensed but are on hand)
- Information about liabilities or contingent liabilities, such as equipment leases you pay monthly (but don't show as a debt on your balance sheet) or potential claims against the practice for services performed in the past

Overall, this is your chance to tell the appraiser what makes your practice unique, so don't miss this opportunity by assuming that the appraiser will know enough to ask you all the right questions. Speak up!

or she cannot ensure similar results in the future. The objective is to use historical operating results as the basis for determining future profits. To do so, the valuator must decide what adjustments should be made to historical numbers when arriving at adjusted earnings.

Taxing Matters

Financial statements are prepared primarily to provide the data needed for filing income tax returns. As a result, the financial statements are the result of the tax elections that the practice made in the past. For example, one practice may choose to record income at the time the services are performed, while another records income only when the client pays the bill. The latter approach (the cash method of accounting discussed later in this chapter) may defer the reporting of taxable income and the payment of income taxes, but for appraisal purposes it understates the value of the services the practice has provided to its clients. During step 6 of the appraisal process, when your appraiser is adjusting the historical information of the business, he or she will take these differences in accounting methods into consideration.

Similarly, if your practice shows profits for the year to date and you discuss year-end tax planning with your accountant, you may well be advised to accelerate payments for drug and supply expenses into the current year. This move may reduce current income tax and may therefore provide temporary or even permanent tax savings. For appraisal purposes, however, the only visible effect will be an increase in the supplies expense, which by itself would not necessarily alert the appraiser to what actually happened.

If the hospital's financial statements are compared from year to year for differences in income and expense items (called a "flux review"), then the appraiser may notice that the supplies expense is higher in one year and lower in the next. That may trigger a question to you. Certainly, if the appraiser is trying to determine normalized expected earnings, then he or she must analyze these tax-related swings in income or expenses if they are material.

Be sure to let your appraiser know if adjustments were made for taxes, which might affect the historical information he or she has been given.

An appraiser will deal with the issues below in analyzing your practice's financial information. While this list is not all-inclusive, it should provide you with a basic understanding of the types of adjustments the appraiser may make and the rationale behind those adjustments. Keep in mind that what is not on the financial statements is sometimes as important as what is. When making adjustments, the appraiser may add expense categories, change the amount of an expense item, or ignore certain items altogether. If you don't understand the adjustments being made, ask the appraiser to explain them.

Additional Items to Consider When Analyzing Financial Statements

Reviewing financial statements requires a bit of knowledge and a lot of common sense. Even a nonfinancial person can identify numbers that seem unreasonable. Each asset and liability on the balance sheet should be analyzed to be sure that the numbers make sense. For example, liability accounts with a negative value often mean that payments have not been recorded properly.

Similarly, income and expense numbers should be reviewed in light of the reader's knowledge of how veterinary practices operate. Numbers that seem too high or too low merit additional follow-up, as do accounts that are not clearly identified and properly labeled.

Finally, reports from the hospital's practice-management software can provide additional information about revenue, production by service category, and information about new and continuing clients that is likely not included anywhere in the practice's profit-and-loss statement. Items that might require adjustment include the following:

- *Expenses as a percentage of gross revenue:* There are resources available in the profession to compare one practice's key expenses with those of other practices. AAHA publishes *Financial & Productivity Pulsepoints*, which is an excellent source of these data. Percentages for a practice that seem either high or low likely suggest the need for further investigation. On one hand, the difference may be merely the result of classifying expenses differently; on the other, there may be substantive variations in the practice's expense structure.

- *Doctor compensation as a percentage of doctor production:* Most practices track production by doctor and by service code as well as average transaction charge (ATC, also called average client transaction, ACT) and the number of transactions. These data can be compared with data from other practices for reasonableness.

- *Facility rent:* When practice owners also own the real estate, they generally set the rent to approximate the underlying mortgage payment as well as real estate taxes and insurance. This amount may be significantly higher or lower than market rent for the facility. Buyers of the practice need to know what rent they will be paying for the same facility, so it may be helpful to ask a commercial real estate expert to provide a determination of fair rent.

- *Inventory:* Is the inventory undervalued? Overvalued? Obsolete? What's included in the figure? When was a physical count last taken? It is a danger sign when the same number is on the books for inventory for consecutive years. This indicates that no count was done and that the number is an estimate. This is still fairly common in small practices that do not use practice management software to track inventory.

- *Intangibles:* Intangibles such as trademarks, patents, covenants not to compete, and goodwill should be stated at current economic value. An appraiser must be careful not to count both purchased goodwill and computed current goodwill as assets. Also, a covenant not to compete resulting from an earlier purchase may still be carried on the books even though the term of the restriction has long since expired.

- *Accounts receivable and accounts payable:* What do the clients owe the practice, and what are the practice's outstanding debts that should be on the balance sheet (for example, unpaid expenses)? Is there an aged list of accounts receivable? Are they actively being collected? Are they part of the assets being sold or purchased? Does the practice track its outstanding amounts due to vendors on its financial statements? Should those payables be included in the valuation as a reduction of the value of the equity?

- *Allowance for bad debts:* If there is an allowance, is the allowance adequate? Should some of the accounts receivable be written off? Because additions to the allowance are not deductible for tax purposes, most practices do not estimate uncollectible accounts and instead carry their receivables at the full amount until they are collected or written off. This can result in receivables from several years ago still being shown as assets, even though no collection efforts are in process that would suggest the cash will ever come in.

- *Fixed assets:* How have they been depreciated? Is the list of furniture and equipment complete? Does it match what is actually in the practice as well as what is shown on the depreciation schedule?

- *Loans from the owner* (where the cash went from the owner to the practice): Should these be reclassified as owners' equity, or will the practice actually repay the owner with interest? Has interest been paid? Is there a promissory note?

- *Loans to the owner* (where the cash went from the practice to the owner): Does the owner plan to repay the debt to the practice with interest, or should this be reclassified as compensation? Has the amount changed over time? Is interest being paid? Is there a promissory note?

Cash or Accrual Statements

It is not always apparent from the statement of income or expenses whether the income is being reported as it is earned or when clients actually pay for the services. If income is recorded when it is earned (when the service is performed), the statements are said to be prepared on the accrual method of accounting. If income is recorded only when the cash is received, they are said to be prepared on the cash, or income tax, method. Many professional practices use the cash method for income tax purposes to avoid paying tax on fees they have not yet received. But even if that is the case, the monthly financial statements may still be on the accrual method. In this case the balance sheet should show accounts receivable in the asset section.

For most practices, unpaid client accounts are small and fairly current. Therefore, the practice's gross income might not be significantly different no matter which

More Taxing Matters

Q: Can I use a different accounting method on my financial statements than on my tax return?

A: U.S. tax law allows practices to keep their internal financial statements on the accrual method (showing accounts receivable and payable) while reporting profit and loss on the tax return using the cash method. In those situations, the practice's tax preparer converts the books from accrual to cash as part of the tax-preparation process at year-end. This defers revenue and may therefore defer income taxes. But for those practices that have higher unpaid expenses than uncollected receivables at year-end, reporting on the cash method for tax purposes can actually accelerate income. Certain larger practices are required to use the accrual method under current U.S. tax law. See your tax preparer if you are unsure which method of accounting you are or should be using.

Q: Should I treat my inventory as an asset on my financial statements?

A: Sometimes practices use the cash method of accounting, hoping to avoid having to account for their inventory (pharmaceuticals and retail items like food and leashes). As a result, they make large purchases of drugs and supplies at year-end, planning to deduct the entire cost in the current year. Normal accounting procedures would suggest that the cost of those large purchases should be deducted in the following year when the practice generates the revenue associated with those purchases, which is a better matching of income and expenses. Most accountants do agree, however, that medical supplies, such as sutures or anesthesia, that you use in providing services, but don't generally sell directly to the client, are properly deducted in the year they are acquired and do not need to be counted as part of your inventory for income tax purposes. Be sure the appraiser has information about the current cost of the inventory and supply items on hand, since you definitely want them to be included in the overall value of the practice.

method is used, especially over a period of several years. Nevertheless, the appraiser needs to know which method was used in the financial statements you provide.

The same theory holds true for the recording of expenses. With the accrual method, an account called "accounts payable" will generally appear on the balance sheet in the liability section. The balance in this account represents the sum of expenses the practice has incurred but that have not yet been paid as of the date of the financial statements. On the cash basis, an expense is recorded only when it is paid and never appears as a debt on the balance sheet. If expenses are recorded when they are paid rather than when the invoice is received, it is impossible to tell from the face of the financial statements whether there are significant unpaid expenses. These unrecorded liabilities could significantly affect the value of the practice, since actual expenses could well be understated, particularly during a cash crunch.

One of the most common errors in valuations of veterinary practices is to ignore the impact of cash versus accrual accounting. If the practice uses cash accounting, so that accounts receivable are not recorded on the balance sheet, the value of those receivables should be added to practice revenue and value. Frequently, there is no mention of accounts receivable at all. Even though the amount may be small and the net change from year to year minimal, it is very relevant to buyer and seller. They will need to determine who gets to keep the money when these fees are eventually collected, and disclosing them in the valuation report facilitates that discussion. Similarly, unpaid expenses that are not recorded on the balance sheet can distort the practice's value. If these unpaid expenses are not disclosed, true profits may be overstated. Unpaid expenses can be material, especially in distressed or troubled practices that are short of cash.

As you might suspect, there are hybrid methods of accounting as well. What is important for the appraisal is that the valuator determine exactly how and when the practice records income and expenses. Regardless of whether the valuation report is prepared on the cash or accrual method, be sure the same method is used throughout the valuation report to avoid under- or overreporting of assets or net income, either of which can affect the valuation result.

Unrecorded Assets

If the practice owns life insurance policies on the owners' lives, and the policy provides for a cash surrender value, that amount should show as an asset on the financial statements. However, many small practices do not record this asset. Appraisers will often ask the owners for this information, but if your appraiser does not ask, you should volunteer it. Otherwise, it may be overlooked.

Supplies and small items of equipment that are expensed when purchased, rather than carried as assets, are also frequently overlooked. There may be other assets that need to be recorded on the appraiser's adjusted balance sheet as well, such as goodwill (discussed below), prepaid expenses, patient lists, trade names, and favorable leases. These items should be added to the recorded assets if the appraiser determines that they are material to the calculation or conclusion of value.

Nonoperating Assets

Sometimes the opposite is true: that is, assets appear on the financial statements but they are not part of the normal practice operations. These assets are called "nonoperating assets." Practice operations and profits do not depend on having these items in the practice.

For example, many practice owners have the practice purchase their personal vehicle, even though they may use it only infrequently for business purposes. (Of course, ambulatory equine or food-animal practices may legitimately have vehicles owned and used exclusively within the practice.) Alternatively, some practices retain cash in the practice accounts as they save for particular purposes such as the down payment on land for a new facility.

Valuators usually set the nonoperating assets aside in calculating the value of the practice. They add in nonoperating assets at the end of the process, however, if they will actually be retained in the practice or become part of the ownership transition.

Owners' Compensation

An appraiser must determine both how owners are paid and whether or not the amount is reasonable. This requires some detective work, as many owners of closely held companies are quite creative in the way they compensate themselves. Sadly, some of the methods they use, including a few of those mentioned below, are illegal or unethical.

Although some tax-saving techniques are clearly wrong, much tax planning falls into the "grey zone," that is, aggressive but still allowable under current law. We mention these practices not to make recommendations about compensation but to recognize the reality that these situations exist and that they do affect the valuation. Often they reduce the value of the business, so that a business owner who thought he or she was getting a tax break or extra income ultimately ends up suffering a loss.

Upon the advice of their accountants, for example, owners may be renting real estate or equipment to the practice at rents that are artificially high or low. They may be running travel, entertainment, education, and automobile expenses through the clinic that are not totally related to the practice. They may also have legitimate fringe benefit plans that pay child care or medical expenses with pretax dollars— which means they do not show up on the owners' W-2 forms as wages at the end of the year. Some owners barter with their clients, exchanging services with no cash changing hands. Bartering is fine, so long as both parties report the resulting income and deduct only expenses that are allowable under current tax law.

Not legitimate are businesses where the practice pays some of the owners' personal expenses, such as utilities or supplies, which get buried in the practice's expense accounts. Even worse, there are still some practices that do not record all their income because the owner takes the cash directly without running it through the practice's records. If your practice is doing this, or if you are looking to buy a practice that has done this in the past, be very careful. Not only is this illegal and easily discoverable by the taxing authorities, but it makes it much more difficult for the valuator to determine what the actual income and actual expenses were.

If you are the seller, don't expect a buyer to take on faith your assertion that the practice profits are really greater than they appear because you pocketed a good portion of the cash. If you are willing to risk penalties and even jail time by cheating the government, why would a buyer think you would be totally honest with him or her? You may think you saved some taxes, but your practice sale will net you less than if you had kept an accurate set of books over the years.

If an owner uses questionable or illegal techniques to reduce taxable income, the appraiser is put in an uncomfortable situation. Data given to a valuator are confidential, and the appraiser will not disclose it to any other person or agency unless compelled by law to do so. Situations can arise, however, where a disgruntled employee or an unsuccessful buyer might cause that kind of information to fall into the hands of a taxing authority. Therefore, the owner takes a risk by using those techniques and then expecting an appraiser to document them for purposes of increasing practice value. Language in the report explaining the owner's techniques in order to add back personal expenses or report previously unreported income may be dangerous. A far better approach is to avoid those techniques in the first place, as there are worse fates than paying taxes.

One or more owners may have a spouse or child on the payroll who may or may not be providing services equivalent to the salary received. Sometimes this is a way to increase family income and provide retirement benefits to an otherwise non-working spouse. Sometimes owners have a parent on the payroll in order to supplement the parent's retirement income. If you are doing this, be sure to disclose this information to the valuator. The valuator will need to know whether the salary is legitimate and what services are actually being performed. On the other hand, many spouses provide significant services to the practice and are fairly compensated, or even underpaid, for the work they do, including some who receive no compensation at all. Determining the facts in each situation is important in calculating true practice profits.

Some owners choose to take part of their compensation in the form of expense reimbursements for travel or entertainment expenses, while others choose to be paid only wages that show on the W-2 form at year-end. Owners may be paying insurance premiums for themselves, excessive continuing education costs, or significant contributions to pension or retirement plans through the practice. Even in the same practice, two owners may be getting compensated in very different ways. Different amounts on their W-2 forms do not necessarily mean that the owners are compensated unequally, merely that they are paid differently.

If the owners' compensation is buried in the financial statements in any of these ways, then practice profits will appear to be lower on the face of the statements. Because of U.S. tax regulations related to personal service corporations, veterinary practices that want to avoid the maximum federal income tax rate for regular, or C, corporations are becoming more creative at using deductions to reduce taxable income. These amounts still represent owners' compensation for valuation purposes, however, and are part of the cash flow generated by the practice.

An appraiser can detect these practices only by reviewing historical financial information and talking to the owners. Locating and modifying net income for these items may require significant adjustment to the recorded earnings to decide what normalized profits really are. (See sidebar "Items That Might Represent Additional Owners' Compensation," for some of the items that may be disguised owners' compensation for purposes of the valuation.)

Retirement Plans

A wide variety of retirement plans now exist in veterinary practices, though the most common are 401(k) plans and SIMPLE IRA plans. Both types have features allowing the employee to contribute to the plan through payroll withholding and also require

Items That Might Represent Additional Owners' Compensation

Owners of closely held businesses, including veterinary practices, are adept at taking income out of the business in ways designed to reduce income taxes. One of the most common techniques is to take it in the form of perquisites, or "perks." These are expenses that may or may not be business-related but are paid by the practice and expensed on the company's books.

Amounts deemed to be perks should be added back to the practice's profits in determining adjusted earnings *if they will not continue.* If you are buying only a piece of a practice, you must find out whether there will be any changes in the items listed below. Unless you are buying 100% of the practice or will have the controlling interest on the board of directors of a corporation, will become the managing member of a limited liability company, or will become the general partner with control of operations in a partnership, these practices may not change after you buy in. Unless you have control, be sure these items are governed by an agreement among owners or by employment contracts before you become an owner.

Following is a list of the more common perks used in veterinary practices. While some of these are valid business expenses, they are still discretionary, since not all owners in all practices would have similar expenses. (No judgment as to the ethical or tax issues involved in these expenses is implied.)

- Non-business entertainment, meals, country club dues, health club dues, and related expenditures
- Automobiles owned or leased by the practice but used by the owner for personal purposes or by the owner's spouse; also the related expenses of operating such vehicles
- Personal use of business credit cards and company checks for personal office supplies, postage, etc.
- Home computers listed as practice assets
- Trading veterinary services for personal goods or services
- Medical and health care costs not covered by insurance but paid by the practice
- Life and disability insurance premiums
- Pension or profit-sharing contributions to the owner(s)' accounts in retirement plans that are designed to provide significant benefits to certain classes of employees
- Non-business gifts
- Personal use of boats, airplanes, horse trailers, and the like

continues >

Items That Might Represent Additional Owners' Compensation, *continued*

- Personal expenses related to owners' residences, including lawn maintenance or snow removal, telephone, Internet access, cell phones, electricity, and water
- Pet food, pet care, kennel costs, and boarding for personal animals
- Maid and cleaning services at personal residences
- Purchase of personal furniture and clothing as supplies

- Personal landscaping and house repairs
- College tuition for children, spouses, or employees
- Nonworking family members on the payroll
- Legal and accounting fees for personal items, including personal tax return preparation, financial planning, or will preparation
- Vacation or other travel expenses classified as continuing education costs

the practice to make a contribution on the employee's behalf. The actual rules are governed by the plan documents themselves, so valuators must understand the kind of retirement plan in place and how it is operating in the practice.

Most valuators now view company contributions to nonowners' retirement accounts as ongoing operating expenses and do not add them back as discretionary or nonrecurring expenses. Contributions made on behalf of the owner(s) are an exception to this rule, since the owners can generally choose whether or not to participate themselves. Sometimes specific retirement plans are adopted because the plan can be designed to allow the owners and/or doctors to set aside substantial retirement funds while providing a fairly small benefit for the other eligible employees.

If the assets of the practice are being sold, the current retirement plan will likely be terminated, with the buyer adopting a new plan, if any, of his or her choosing. In the case of associate buy-ins, however, it's important for the parties to determine whether the existing plan will continue as is or if there will be modifications to it as the result of the new ownership.

Unrecorded Liabilities

During the life of a practice, situations can arise that create liabilities, such as malpractice claims, employee disputes, or contract issues. A purchaser of the practice needs to be aware of any potential claims against the practice and should get representation from the seller that full disclosure of these potential liabilities has been made. Attorneys generally recommend that the buyer ask the seller to indemnify the purchaser from any such exposure.

If the potential liabilities are significant and, in the appraiser's view, may become actual debts of the practice, they need to be calculated or estimated. Unless some other provision is made, they may reduce the value of the practice. In an equity purchase (an associate buy-in, for example), unrecorded liabilities will be assumed automatically by the purchaser in the absence of a written agreement to the contrary.

Fixed Assets

Furniture, fixtures, and equipment are usually carried on the practice's books at original cost less accumulated depreciation. This figure may be higher or lower than actual value and should be converted to a reasonable approximation of the current market value of these assets.

If furniture, fixtures, and equipment represent a large portion of a practice's assets and a precise value is necessary, an appraiser who deals in this type of property can be hired to provide estimates for the veterinary practice appraiser. It can be costly to take this route, however, and it is rarely worth going to the extra expense. For most practices, an approximation of value based on the practice's fixed asset records will be close enough to satisfy both buyers and sellers, particularly if the valuator is using a single-period or discounted future earnings approach.

One acceptable method is to compute replacement cost reduced to a figure representing the value over the remaining economic life of the asset (see sidebar "Estimating the Value of Fixed Assets"). This method enables the appraiser to place a value on fixed assets that are still in use but are fully depreciated, on fixed assets that were written off in the years in which they were purchased, and on fixed assets that simply never appeared on the books.

In recent years, income tax authorities have allowed businesses to write off much larger sums for furniture and equipment

---

Estimating the Value of Fixed Assets

An appraiser may reduce the replacement cost of a fixed asset to a figure representing the value over the remaining economic life of the asset. For example, if a piece of equipment that cost $2,100 eight years ago has a seven-year life for tax purposes because of the tax rules in effect when it was purchased, then its book value now is zero, since it is fully depreciated. However, if its expected useful life is ten years and it would cost $3,000 to buy a new one, then its value to the practice is $600. This is computed by taking the replacement cost of the asset ($3,000) and reducing it by 80%, since eight of the ten years of its economic life have passed. The net adjustment, therefore, would be to add $600 to the stated book value of the practice's fixed assets.

---

in the year acquired, rather than claiming depreciation deductions (expensing a portion of the cost) for these assets over five or seven years. This is an annual tax election that is made by many practices to reduce income taxes in the current year.

For valuation purposes, however, adjustments will be needed, since the book value of the assets will be zero. In addition, although it is not correct accounting, many practices struggle to track their fixed assets properly over the years and may be unable to produce an accurate list of what is actually in use in the practice as of the valuation date.

The appraiser must adjust not only for assets that are still in use but not on the books, but also for assets that are still on the books but no longer in the practice. Even though equipment is broken or lost, owners often forget to tell their tax preparer, with the result that the financial statements still reflect the costs of items that are long gone. For this reason, valuators frequently ask for a current list of equipment and furniture on hand and then compare this list with the depreciation schedule prepared as part of the tax preparation process. Differences then generate questions to reconcile the two lists.

Equipment Leases

Equipment leases are very common in the veterinary profession. Rather than buying a piece of equipment, practices can choose to lease it under a contract between the vendor (or a related lender) and the practice. During the term of the lease, most practices simply record the payments as expenses. The equipment is not listed as an asset and the remaining portion of the lease is not listed as a liability.

However, often the lease contract allows the practice to purchase the equipment at the end of the lease term for an amount as small as $1. Not surprisingly, the IRS, for income tax purposes, views these leases as disguised purchases, since all the facts about the transaction are known up front. If the lease contract calls for a payment at the end of the lease term that is based on fair market value of the equipment at that time, then the payments are considered rent for the use of the equipment, not payments to buy it. In that case, even though the payments were properly expensed, they will not continue indefinitely and should not be treated as an ongoing normal practice expense beyond the end of the lease term.

The leases that are considered purchases by the IRS likely do not show up as liabilities on the financial statements, even though the practice is obligated to make these payments in the future. Some tax preparers properly reclassify this kind of lease as the purchase of an asset with an offsetting liability for the stream of payments, but many do not. Therefore, it's important for the appraiser to get information about any equipment leases. He or she needs to see how the practice has accounted for them historically. When a practice is being sold, many equipment vendors will allow buyers to assume these leases under the same terms as those already in force for the seller. Alternatively, in a buyout situation, it may be better for the seller simply to pay off the lease.

The Practice Facility

The practice facility and other real property owned by the practice should be appraised separately, since most business appraisers are not also real estate appraisers.

The value of real estate owned by the practice is undoubtedly material to the valuation of the practice as a whole. Commercial real estate appraisers have observed that appraising veterinary clinic facilities can be very difficult and expensive, since there are few comparable properties selling in a particular locale. In addition, the value of the property will vary significantly depending on whether it is being valued as an existing clinic or for a different future use. Once again, good communication with the appraiser is necessary, as the exact way that the real estate appraisal affects the practice appraisal depends to a great extent on what the practice owners' plans are for the property. Keep in mind that the practice owners may own the facility in a separate legal entity, not within the practice itself.

The practice owners may not be interested in selling the real estate along with the practice. Sometimes, the owners prefer to rent the facility to the buyer by entering into a lease agreement, generally with an option for the buyer of the practice to purchase the facility at some point in the future. The rent the practice will pay will affect the valuation of the practice because it will have an impact on its future earnings. Therefore, it is important for the appraiser to know what the terms of the lease will be. Practice sellers who continue to own the real estate must understand that it may not be possible to get top dollar for the practice itself if the future rent is set artificially high or is more than the practice can reasonably afford to pay.

One other possibility is that the facility has been leased from an unrelated third party, but the practice has spent thousands or even hundreds of thousands of dollars to build out the space and make it a functioning veterinary hospital. From a valuation standpoint, there are two problems here. First, if the buyer cannot assume the existing lease but has to negotiate a lease with the landlord, the terms of the new lease may affect future practice profits, and therefore the value of the practice. Second, from a legal point of view, those costs to build out the space have value only so long as the practice occupies that space. At the end of the lease, those leasehold improvements revert to the building's owner. With the exception of items that can be removed easily, they will stay in the building. If a buyer plans to relocate the practice in the near future, the leasehold improvements have limited value to that purchaser, even though the practice may have paid a great deal for them.

Sometimes the practice's financial statements show no rent expense at all. This can happen when the practice has a single owner who also owns the facility and does not pay rent for its use. This situation artificially inflates the practice profits on paper. However, when ownership changes, the seller is not likely to give the buyer rent-free use of the facility, so the appraiser must determine what rent the seller expects to charge the new practice owner. Alternatively, if the facility is being sold along with the practice, the new owner will have to set aside other funds to service the debt to buy the facility. Either way, the use of the facility will be an ongoing practice expense.

Therefore, the valuator must inquire as to the ownership of the facility, its current market value (if it will be sold), and the rent the buyer will pay to occupy that space.

Goodwill

Goodwill continues to be the most troublesome area in business valuation. If two appraisers disagree significantly over the value of a practice, it will probably be due to disagreements in this area.

"Goodwill" is a generic term used to describe a practice's intangible assets. Unless a practice was purchased in the past and part of the purchase price was allocated to goodwill at that time, this asset will not show on the financial statements. Nevertheless, it may be the most valuable asset in the practice. Goodwill includes the value of the practice as a going concern (the value of having the equipment, patient list, staff, and so on already assembled and functioning); the reputation of the hospital and its doctors within the community; the right to practice veterinary medicine; and perhaps the opportunity to work in one or more specialties.

In addition, for goodwill to have value to a buyer, it must be transferable— that is, it must stay with the practice when the seller(s) walk out the door. For that reason, most buyers will only consider purchasing a practice when the seller(s) provide a covenant not to compete as part of the contract terms. The duration and the geographic area covered vary, depending on the practice and the locale. Keep in mind that these covenants are enforceable under the law when they are related to a purchase/sale, even though non-compete agreements in employment contracts (between owners and nonowner employees) may not be valid under local law. Transferability of goodwill is discussed in more detail below.

Goodwill in other types of businesses tends to be easier to quantify than goodwill in professional practices. With other types of businesses, earnings over and above a normal rate of return, or earnings in excess of industry averages, may indicate goodwill. Goodwill in professional practices is much more complex. Separating the goodwill of the professional practice from the goodwill of the professional person can be difficult, or even impossible, to achieve. Nevertheless, goodwill has value only if the seller can transfer it to the buyer. Following are some of the factors involved.

Practice Goodwill and Professional Goodwill

Practice goodwill is value that is associated with the business or entity, whereas professional goodwill is value associated with the individual veterinarian. In a valuation, the assumption is that the seller(s) will transfer both kinds of goodwill, and little or no effort is made to distinguish between them. However, sometimes the actual purchase documents will state separate values for each, generally because of differences in income tax treatment among various kinds of practice entities.

Transferring Goodwill

Even if expected earnings are calculated and used to compute a value for goodwill that is included in the practice's overall value, the question is whether this goodwill belongs to the practice or to the owner(s). If you are the potential buyer, it makes a great deal of difference to you if this goodwill will leave with the seller or will remain for you to enjoy. It is these earnings related to goodwill that create the cash flow to enable the purchaser to pay the seller (or repay the lender) for the practice.

Most buyers today are unwilling to take a significant salary reduction to fund the purchase of a veterinary practice and so must rely on the practice's earnings to do so. Therefore, maintaining the goodwill and the earnings it represents is critical to the buyer's success. Likewise, it is critical to the seller that the buyer be able to make the scheduled payments. No one wants to see their practice fall into disrepair or fail because the buyer can't generate enough profits to make the payments to buy the practice.

In a perfect world, all buyers would borrow money from outside sources to buy a practice so the sellers would receive only cash up front. In the real world, however, many sellers end up financing at least a portion of the purchase price to reduce the primary lender's risk. Therefore, if the earnings in the practice after the sale do not support the price paid, the buyer either will be strapped financially or will default on the purchase. Neither of these situations benefits buyer or seller. To help ensure success, the previous owner frequently takes specific steps to ease the transition.

One of the best ways to preserve goodwill in a practice during a change of ownership is for the seller to continue to provide services during a transitional period (perhaps three to six months on a part-time basis). In this way, he or she can introduce the new owner to clients and help to provide continuity of patient care. Generally, sellers

A Plan for Maintaining Goodwill

When a new doctor takes over a veterinary practice, clients may decide that it's time for a change and go elsewhere. Without a well-planned, thoughtful transition process, a practice can quickly lose much of the goodwill that was built up over the years. To avoid this and retain goodwill when the practice changes hands, buyer and seller should negotiate a plan whereby the former doctor will stay on for a few months, perhaps part-time, to introduce established clients to the new doctor. Clients are more likely to stay with the practice if the old doctor recommends the new one. The plan should be put in writing and signed by both parties, both referenced in the purchase/sales agreement and included in a separate employment or independent contractor agreement.

Buyers must understand that once the seller leaves the area or is otherwise unable to be in the practice, the goodwill begins eroding immediately. Having the buyer work in the practice prior to the sale, if feasible, can help introduce clients to the new doctor. Introducing the new doctor on the practice's website can ease the transition as well.

don't make good associates over the long run, since it is hard to go from controlling the practice to working for someone who now owns it. However, having buyer and seller work together during a transition period can benefit everyone, including the clients. If this kind of plan will be in place, the buyer and seller are well advised to negotiate the terms of the plan and put them in writing. In particular, they must be very specific about the compensation and benefits, if any, that the practice will pay the former owner, as well as the services expected and the term of this arrangement.

In the absence of this kind of planned transition, it can be very difficult to transfer goodwill, especially in a one-person practice. Veterinarians often observe that client loyalty is not as strong as it was in the past. If the client's loyalty is to the individual veterinarian, a new doctor taking over the same practice may not be able to retain that client. The chances are excellent that the client has been bombarded with information about the competition and has heard good things from friends and business associates about at least one of the practice's competitors.

If, in the normal course of business, the client can be introduced to the new doctor by the old doctor, it is much more likely that the client will stay with the practice. This is because the new owner is now someone he or she has met and who was, in effect, recommended by the current veterinarian.

Impact of Risk in Calculating the Value of Goodwill

For veterinary practices, goodwill is often quantified by capitalizing the practice's earnings, though there are different ways to make that calculation. This will be discussed in the case study as we explore three different valuation methods, all of which use an income approach as part of the calculation of goodwill and overall practice value (see Chapter 7).

Goodwill in a professional practice comes from the presence of those factors that cause repeat business and that are intangible in nature. Quantifying goodwill allows a prospective buyer to distinguish one practice from another based on the likelihood of attaining similar or greater levels of profitability by owning and operating the practice.

For years there was an underlying belief that a 20% capitalization rate was appropriate in all veterinary practice valuations, and that rate was used extensively in calculating goodwill. However, logic would say that a practice in a depressed geographical area with declining profitability has to be more risky than a practice in a growing community with increasing gross revenue and profits each year. Because of the higher risk involved in transferring a business in a depressed area, the first practice has to be worth less than the second, all other factors being equal. The factors listed in the sidebar "Factors in Veterinary Practice Goodwill" can help valuators think through the comparative risk of one practice versus another, resulting in more accurate practice valuations.

Capitalization Rates and
Discount Rates

Part of the complexity of valuing goodwill is determining and applying appropriate capitalization or discount rates. In the very simplest terms, valuations of veterinary practices depend on determining the expected earnings from the practice and then applying a capitalization or discount rate that properly reflects the risk of generating those earnings as well as the buyer's expected rate of return.

Experience has shown that if you ask a group of veterinarians what rate of return they expect from their investment in a veterinary practice, you will get a wide range of answers. Some argue that the work itself is reward enough, as they love what they do and would continue to practice as a veterinarian even if they didn't get paid at all. (Those are rare, though.) A greater number focus their efforts on patient care and let the business side of the practice take care of itself, resulting in wide variations in levels of profitability. Others see veterinary practices as high-risk businesses; they

Factors in Veterinary Practice Goodwill

Several years ago, the Veterinary Valuation Resource Council of VetPartners, a nonprofit association of veterinary consultants and advisers, identified thirteen factors that should be analyzed in determining the value of a veterinary practice and its goodwill:

- Growth in adjusted profitability
- Ability to effectively transfer goodwill
- Revenue growth
- Location
- Quality of staff
- Demand for services
- Facility
- Demographics
- Practice stability
- Competitive environment
- Lease terms
- Effective management systems
- Desirability and marketability

These factors all reinforce the fact that no two practices are alike and no two practices have the same degree of inherent risk. For more information on these risk factors, contact the Veterinary Valuation Resource Council of VetPartners at www.vetpartners.org. Overall, the first two factors and the last one are especially important.

Estimating Profitability

If you are unsure how the estimated adjusted profitability in a given practice compares with that of others in the profession, go to www.ncvei.org, the website of the National Commission on Veterinary Economic Issues, and complete the VetPartners/NCVEI Profitability Estimator. There are specific tools for estimating profitability in wellness, specialty/emergency referral, and equine practices. These tools are based on "The No-Lo Practice: Avoiding a Practice Worth Less," created by the Veterinary Valuation Resource Council of VetPartners and published in *Veterinary Economics* in 2007.

expect to be paid for their services, however, and to receive a return on their investment as high as 25% or 30% per year.

With the growth of corporate consolidators, the focus on return on investment is becoming more pronounced in the industry. Although profits are not the only factor impacting practice value, they are a significant component. There are exceptions, but it is generally safe to assume that practices with higher profitability will have a higher value at the end of the appraisal process and will command a higher price in actual sales transactions. Conversely, practices with lower profitability will usually have a lower value and command a lower price.

Because the determination of the capitalization rate has such a major impact on the calculation of practice value, you should expect a valuator to be able to discuss how he or she determined this rate. The valuation literature is full of opinions about how to develop these rates, and there is no one way that works for all practices. However, the valuator should be able to explain how the rate was determined, as well as how the business being valued ranks in terms of risk when compared with other practices. Assessing risk is a subjective process and accounts for a great deal of the variation in value of the same practice among different appraisers.

Valuing Specialty Referral and Emergency Practices

In the past couple of decades, a number of referral practices have been created around the country. Some of these started as emergency practices owned by a group of veterinarians who wanted to provide quality care during their clients' emergencies without being on call on nights and weekends. At the same time, many veterinarians have chosen to specialize in a particular area, creating both stand-alone and mobile practices offering specific kinds of services. Also, groups of specialists have congregated and formed specialty referral centers providing a wider range of specialty services under one roof. General-practice veterinarians refer clients and patients to these practices to handle diagnostics or care that go beyond what the general practitioner is prepared or willing to handle.

There are special issues involved in valuing a referral practice. Each of these practices is unique because of the specific mix of services provided. It's important that the appraiser for such a practice understand the differences between wellness and referral practices, that he or she is prepared to make the appropriate adjustments to earnings, and that he or she knows what risk factors need to be taken into account in determining the capitalization or discount rate.

Here are some of the factors that make valuations of specialty referral and emergency practices particularly challenging:

- *Who is the client?* Referral practices have two distinct groups of clients. One is referring veterinarians, who are generally the primary source of the cases they see. The other is, of course, the animals' owners.

- *Who develops and maintains the relationship?* The referral practice staff must be able to work effectively with these referring doctors and develop personal relationships with them.

- *Who is responsible for communication with the referring veterinarian (rDVM)?* Referral practices must have systems in place for providing complete and timely communication about each case's progress to the referring doctor, and they must make sure that each case is returned promptly to the referring veterinarian for future work, so that the rDVM doesn't feel at risk of losing clients by making the referral.

- *Who is responsible for communication with the animal's owner?* The communication skills of the referral practice staff must be excellent at making complex medical facts and jargon understandable to animal owners, and they must be skilled at explaining medical options, some of which are very difficult and emotionally painful for clients to accept.

- *What equipment and facilities are expected to be in place?* Specialty practices are expected to have state-of-the-art facilities and equipment, and their doctors and staff must present a professional image at all times. The purchase or lease of expensive medical equipment is therefore a necessity, as is excellent staff training.

- *Can goodwill be transferred?* Transferring goodwill can be particularly challenging with these practices, since a boarded surgeon cannot easily step into the shoes of a dermatologist or an ophthalmologist. This results in a shorter list of potential buyers, which increases the risk of transferring ownership quickly and efficiently.

- *What impact does the overall economy have on referrals?* These practices are more vulnerable to changes in the overall economy, since in tough economic times clients cannot afford many of the treatment options available and thus the number of euthanasias increases.

- *Where do clients come from?* These practices capture clients from a large geographic area, so they are more vulnerable to specialty competitors entering the local market. Some metropolitan areas have experienced drops in revenue growth rates and even declines in overall revenue as the number of specialty practices approaches saturation.

- *Can a practice find enough associates and pay them fairly?* The demand for certain specialists has been so high at times that practices must pay above-market compensation to attract strong candidates. This can lead to depressed profits and practice values, unless associates can be persuaded to accept alternative compensation approaches in future years.

- *Are there benchmarks for referral practices?* Average revenue per transaction is higher in referral practices than in wellness practices, but so are the costs. We also know that revenue per transaction varies significantly from one specialty to another. To date, there is little reliable data about referral practices, especially data collected for individual specialties. This makes it more difficult for a valuator to identify what is "normal" in referral practices, thereby making it harder to spot what is unusual about a particular practice.

Valuing Equine, Avian, and Food-Animal Practices

Just as with specialty referral practices, practices specializing in a particular area, such as equine, avian, or food-animal health, present special issues. They operate differently from small-animal practices, and valuators must understand these differences.

Equine and food-animal practices often do a significant amount of field-work, which makes the practice vehicles, as well as the cost to own and operate them, a more significant part of the operations than in practices focusing on small animals. Managing inventory efficiently can also be more of a challenge, since duplicate drugs and supplies may be located simultaneously in several trucks as well as at one or more hospital locations. Often the doctors see many animals at a time during one visit, since the client is actually a barn or a ranch, not necessarily an owner of one animal. Also, the time the doctor spends driving to and from these calls does not directly produce revenue, so the costs to do ambulatory work must be built into the fees for services actually provided. Finally, these clients frequently choose to purchase drugs and supplies from their veterinarian but have on-site personnel to administer them, using the doctor only for unusual situations.

Like other specialty practices, these businesses draw from a larger area than a small-animal practice normally would. In addition, some practices specialize even further, choosing to offer services only in equine reproduction or alternative medicine like acupuncture or rehabilitation, for example.

Avian practices present different issues. Special equipment is needed, such as incubators and gram scales (to measure a bird's weight accurately). In addition, though birds are not large, they are often stressed by travel, so a mobile service may be a valuable part of the practice. Limited data points about avian practice operations and results are available, however, which makes these valuations more challenging than most. As with other specialty practices, the list of potential purchasers is also shorter.

Once you've gathered all the pertinent data and turned it over to your appraiser, he or she will consider all the factors, choose an appropriate method, and conduct an analysis. It will then be time for him or her to write up your report. The next chapter will explain what the report will contain.

6

What to Look for in an Appraisal Report

The engagement letter that is signed by both parties at the beginning of the valuation engagement controls who is entitled to read the report. Because the valuation is done for a specific purpose, and because the value will be different depending on the purpose of the valuation, distribution of the report is restricted. For example, an associate buying 20% of a practice cannot read a report valuing 100% of the practice assets and simply multiply the result by 20% to determine the buy-in price. As discussed previously, the adjustments made in arriving at the appropriate earnings stream will vary depending on whether the buyer will have control or only a minority interest. Therefore, the engagement letter (and the resulting report) will likely limit the use of the report.

Even so, the appraisal report will be read by different people with very different perspectives. First is the person who hired the appraiser, who will be reading it to see if the appraisal makes sense and seems well thought out and fair. Second is one or more potential buyers, who will be reading it to see how it might affect their decision about the purchase. Depending on the purpose of the appraisal, a number of other people may be reading the appraisal report, each with a unique perspective and reasons for being interested.

Everyone will want to know the bottom line. But there are many other items of interest in an appraisal report, and this chapter will provide an overview of these and explain how to interpret the report's finer details. How can you tell if that figure on the bottom line represents the true value of the practice? What does the report say about your chances of making the practice a success once you acquire it? If you are planning a merger, how similar are the operations and accounting methods to the ones in your own practice? To learn the answers to these questions, you need to know how to conduct your own analysis of the report.

In this chapter, we'll assume you are the potential buyer. However, if your actual role is different, read the chapter anyway; you will learn about the main components of an appraisal report and what they mean.

The Report Analysis: An Overview

Before you begin, realize that it will take more than one reading to understand the report fully. In fact, you will want to do some of your own analysis and maybe make a few calculations as well. I would recommend following a multistep process. Here is an overview of how you might approach the project:

Step 1. Read the report from cover to cover.

Step 2. Look for the assumptions that were made and determine whether you agree with these assumptions or would have made different ones.

Step 3. Estimate the mathematical effect of the changes you would have made.

Step 4. Conduct your own analysis of the adjustments made to earnings. Are they reasonable?

Step 5. Look closely at the projected staffing of the practice.

Step 6. Ask the prospective seller for copies of financial statements and tax returns.

Step 7. Do not accept at face value any appraisal that lacks the detail for you to take the steps listed above.

Below we will look in more detail at each of these steps.

Your Step-by-Step Guide
Step 1. Read the Report from Cover to Cover

When you read the appraisal report for the first time, read the entire report from cover to cover, including the charts and lists of numbers. You may be tempted to gloss over complex data and look only for narrative that explains the data. However, by doing so, you will likely miss relevant information.

Even if the data seem complex, careful reading may bring discrepancies or inconsistencies to your attention. These may deserve more follow-up. Don't worry about being unable to understand the entire report. But if you read it all and still don't understand it, you deserve to get an explanation from the appraiser. An appraisal report should be understandable to the average educated person, since the people taking an interest in it are rarely economists or experts in financial matters. If it is difficult to understand, see if you can contact the appraiser directly to get more information. List your questions ahead of time so you can try to get as much done as possible in one meeting or conversation (see sidebar "FAQ: Can Potential Buyers Contact the Appraiser?")

Step 2. Look for the Assumptions and Determine Possible Changes

On second reading, look for the assumptions that were made. There likely will not be a list of stated assumptions, so make notes of your own about the beliefs or theories the appraiser has referenced. You will identify statements about future expectations, adjustments to staffing and expenses, and similar comments that alert you to the appraiser's thoughts.

As discussed earlier, if buyer and seller agree on the assumptions, the range of reasonable values narrows considerably. Therefore, consider what your assumptions would be and how they would be the same or different from the ones made in the report. Do you agree with the assumptions about levels of staffing and any suggested changes to owner, doctor, or staff compensation, for example? If the practice does a lot of boarding, extra staff will be needed to feed, water, and walk the boarded animals; clean the cages; and so on. An appraiser who adjusts staffing costs for such a practice to the same percentage of revenue as for a practice with little or no boarding has made an unreasonable assumption.

FAQ: Can Potential Buyers Contact the Appraiser?

The appraisal report should be written with clarity and geared toward laypeople. A valuation report should give the reader information about what makes the practice unique; it should not simply be a treatise on valuation theory. A full or summary report for a conclusion of value should contain historical background about the practice, information on who owns it currently as well as any changes in ownership over time, and the demographics of the local, regional, and/or national area as of the date of the valuation. The appraiser should explain not only what adjustments were made to historical earnings but also the rationale for making those adjustments. Otherwise, you must simply trust that the adjustments were reasonable and that they were calculated appropriately. In short, by the time you finish reading the report, you should know significantly more about the practice than you did at the beginning.

However, if you are evaluating a practice that you are thinking of buying, but do not yet know a great deal about the practice's finances, you no doubt have a lot of questions, and you may want to contact the appraiser for clarification of complex sections. Your advisers may also want to contact the appraiser directly for clarification of certain items. With the permission of the practice owner (which is generally given), appraisers will frequently discuss their report and the work they did with a serious buyer.

That said, appraisers may be unable to share as much information with you as they could with the party who hired them and still maintain confidentiality about sensitive areas. Also, appraisers do not necessarily want to start at the beginning and explain what's already detailed in the report. In a few cases, you may not be able to talk to the appraiser at all, or you may choose not to do so. In any case, you will need to know how to get the most information that you can from the report itself.

Part of what makes valuations challenging is that no two practices are alike. Trying to adjust every practice's operating results to match some phantom average overlooks the uniqueness of that practice. Look for explanations about the practice's hours of operation, mix of revenue, and the like to see how the facts and figures compare with those of practices where you have worked or that you have observed.

Look particularly at the capitalization or discount rate. As you will see in the case study described in Chapter 7, changing the assumptions that drive these rates changes the numbers significantly. Keep in mind that these rates represent risk, and the risk of generating future profits is always different from one practice to another. These rates must vary from practice to practice, so be wary of rates that simply appear in the report with no explanation at all.

Make sure you know whether the report presents a conclusion of value or a calculation of value (see Chapter 2 for an explanation of how these are different). If it is a calculation report, be sure you agree with the assumptions that were made, which should be clearly stated, since the appraiser did not have free rein to choose the methods and assumptions underlying the valuation result. If it is a conclusion of value report, the appraiser must explain the methods he or she has chosen to use.

Step 3. Estimate the Mathematical Effect of the Changes

If your reading of the report makes you question the valuator's assumptions, take a few minutes to estimate the mathematical effect of the changes you would have made. In some cases, the effect would be minimal. For example, adjusting minor expenses such as postage or laundry up or down will not make much of a difference. On the other hand, lowering the practice's facility rent by thousands of dollars would increase the results of the valuation significantly.

Some appraisers routinely adjust most expenses to their sense of what is normal or reasonable. This habit ignores the variations that make each practice unique. Each practice has its own blend of services, and its operating expenses and many other factors will reflect this. The effect can be either major or minor, depending on the item and the size of the adjustment. If it's major, study the actual numbers further. If the net effect is small, keep reading.

Step 4. Conduct Your Own Analysis of the Earnings

When you look at expected adjusted earnings for the practice, challenge them for reasonableness. Then, if the figures make sense, do your own analysis of how you would spend those earnings. Many appraisal reports attempt to convince you that the practice will be much more profitable in the future than it is currently. Do you agree with that analysis?

Furthermore, has the bottom line already been reduced by owner(s)' compensation, or will your salary come from that figure, along with the dollars to pay off your acquisition loan and to reinvest in new equipment? Are you willing to use the compensation for your services to pay off the loan, or do you expect these funds to come from the practice profits? In other words, most appraisers show the net earnings as funds available for your use, implying that you have already been paid for your services and therefore could take these profits from the practice, either as additional compensation or as profit distributions. However, this is not necessarily true. Which equipment needs to be replaced? Is the staffing adequate? Will you need to remodel or spruce up the clinic to increase efficiency and present the image you want to your clients?

Be sure the profits will be sufficient to pay you a reasonable salary, maintain or grow the practice, make the payments to buy the practice, and still have some cushion for unexpected events. If the profits will not be sufficient, either the price or the payment terms are unreasonable.

Step 5. Look Closely at Projected Staffing

Look very closely at the projected staffing of the practice. If an appraiser wants to increase projected profits in the valuation, one way to do so easily on paper is to argue that the current practice is overstaffed or that the employees have been underperforming. This allows the appraiser to reduce future payroll costs and increase profits accordingly.

However, that assumption may not be reasonable. If the practice is to grow, it may be more likely that doctor and staff costs will increase. Even if the current doctors or staff members are inefficient or unproductive, will they change overnight because you come into the practice? And will your efficiency be at its peak as you get to know the inner workings of the practice and the clients?

Make your own estimate of staffing needs and compare the figures with the ones in the appraisal report.

Step 6. Ask for Copies of Financial Statements and Tax Returns

You can (and should) ask the prospective seller for copies of financial statements and tax returns for your own review. Spot-check the report against these documents to be sure you can trace the relevant numbers. Don't assume that the seller has done this.

Commonly, net income on the financial statements for one or more years is not tied to historical net income in the valuation report. This often occurs because appraisers generally rely on tax return numbers as being most correct, in that they reflect year-end adjustments that the tax preparer made. Also, taxable income is not necessarily the same figure as net income on the financial statements because of the way the figures are presented in the tax return. Even so, there are valuation reports in which the figures are not tied and cannot be reconciled by you or your advisers. If this is the case in the report you are looking at, it is an appropriate question to ask the appraiser. While the differences might not be material, these discrepancies do not increase your confidence in the appraisal and its conclusions about the value. If you start to notice errors, continue checking to see if there are others. If the appraiser was careless in either transferring numbers to the valuation or explaining the differences, you should not trust the report without further investigation.

Step 7. Do Not Accept at Face Value an Appraisal That Lacks Detail

The appraisal report should have sufficient detail for you to take the steps listed above. If it does not, you should not accept its conclusions at face value.

Even if the valuator prepared a short summary report, it should contain information about assumptions and calculations. If not, you should request this from the prospective seller or the appraiser. If it cannot be provided, be skeptical. Taking an appraisal on faith is very risky, and hiring your own appraiser can be expensive. It may be time to look at a different practice.

If, after following these steps and conducting your own analysis of the report, you have obtained a value different from the one reached by the appraiser, you may have room for negotiation with the seller. Presenting your offer with reasons to justify the different numbers may lead to a purchase agreement after all, with some savings for you because you did your homework. If the differences are major, however, and the sale does not take place, you will at least know that you did not make a foolish purchase that might have haunted you for years. Continue looking for the right practice for you, and one that is priced right, and you will eventually succeed.

In the next chapter, we'll look at a case study. So don't make that offer yet. Take the time to see how the process plays out in this detailed example.

Case Study

7

This case study will give you a better understanding of how a valuation might be done for a particular practice. It does not cover every issue that will arise in a practice valuation—nor does it demonstrate the only methods of practice valuation—but it should give you an idea of how an appraiser might conduct an analysis and come to a determination of value. You'll read the facts of a hypothetical practice, see how the appraiser adjusts and examines the financial figures, and learn how the appraiser calculates the value.

Keep in mind that an expected rate of return must be determined for each practice based on the unique characteristics of the practice. The rate used here was chosen for the hypothetical practice discussed based on the facts that I have supplied about the practice, and you must not try to use them for your own practice, which is almost certainly very different from the hypothetical one. Rates also change over time. Even more important, the calculation of a practice's adjusted earnings and capitalization or discount rate must be determined by a skilled and experienced appraiser. When you hire an appraiser, you are buying that judgment and expertise.

The Facts

Dr. Smith, owner and operator of XYZ Animal Hospital, has begun to dream of retirement and longs for the sunny beaches of Florida. Retirement will mean leaving the veterinary practice he built from the ground up and maintained for more than twenty-five years. It is a small-animal practice, and his clientele consists mostly of residents of the nearby neighborhoods. The clinic is located in a busy strip mall in a small northern town and is one of only two clinics within a five-mile radius.

Dr. Smith has employed veterinary technicians and other support staff in the past, but he has never had another doctor in the practice, either as an employee or as an owner. As a result, his hours have increased. He is now working fifty-five to sixty hours per week. He has used a contract relief veterinarian on occasion, but tries to handle the work himself.

He has been making regular contributions to a retirement plan he established for the practice. These assets, when added to his savings, will allow him to retire comfortably if he can get a reasonable price for the practice. It has been a cold winter (it's now January), Florida is beckoning, and Dr. Smith is seriously considering selling the practice in the next twelve months. He decides it is time to hire an appraiser to perform a valuation. If the value is high enough, he will sell. He could probably afford to finance at least a portion of the purchase price to a qualified buyer.

Dr. Smith has already chosen an appraiser based on recommendations and interviews. He has signed an engagement letter and discussed the practice with the appraiser. He believes he has provided all the requested data. This means that steps 1 through 5 of the step-by-step guide outlined in Chapter 2 are already completed. Here is a summary of the outcome for these early stages of the valuation process:

Step 1. Determine the purpose of the valuation: The purpose is to prepare for a sale of the entire practice so that Dr. Smith can retire.

Step 2. Determine if equity or assets are being valued: Because Dr. Smith is selling the entire practice, he will be selling the assets and will be responsible for paying the practice's liabilities from the proceeds of the sale. The only exception would be if the buyer chooses to assume a particular liability, such as an equipment lease or loan.

Step 3. Determine the standard of value: Because this sale will be to an unrelated hypothetical buyer, the appraiser decides that a fair market value standard is appropriate.

Step 4. Establish the effective date of the valuation: The effective date will be December 31, 20x5, the year that just ended. The appraiser has suggested that a potential buyer may want the valuation updated if several months pass between the valuation date and the date of the sale.

Step 5. Gather information: Dr. Smith's accountant has completed the financial statements and tax return for 20x5 and has supplied copies from the previous four years as well. The income statement for the twelve-month period that ended December 31, 20x5, is shown in Table 7.1, and the year-end balance sheet is shown in Table 7.2. The financial statements reflect all year-end adjustments and are tied to the tax returns in all years.

The appraiser has analyzed the financial statements and tax returns for all five years, discovering the following additional facts.

- The practice has increased its income over the past five years by 8% to 12% annually. No specific service or specialty is responsible for the majority of the income, and no change is expected in the structure of services or fees.

- No significant fluctuations in either income or expenses have occurred that distort the financial information and need to be explained. Dr. Smith has answered many questions and has provided additional information in response to the appraiser's questions.

- No material items have come to light so far this year that would impact the practice's financial statements as of the end of last year.

Adjusting the Financial Statements

The appraiser is ready to begin step 6, adjusting the practice's historical financial statements. He'll be using information gained from outside sources (such as statistics collected about veterinary practices by the American Animal Hospital Association and the American Veterinary Medical Association) as well as from Dr. Smith.

Most valuators start by studying historical income and expenses as well as production data for the practice. In this case, the appraiser has found minimal personal items included in the practice's expenses. Adjustments related to these items are reflected in Table 7.3 and will be explained below.

TABLE 7.1   Historical Income Statement

XYZ Animal Hospital, Inc.
Statement of Revenue and Expenses
Income Tax Basis
For the One Month and 12 Months Ended December 31, 20X5

	Current Month	Year to Date	% of Income
INCOME FROM OPERATIONS			
Fees for services	$42,611	$596,297	90.3
Boarding and retail	17,802	64,211	9.7
Total income from operations	60,413	660,508	100.0
COST OF PROFESSIONAL SERVICES			
Drugs and medical supplies	6,844	93,022	14.1
Laboratory costs	1,484	20,870	3.2
Imaging costs	1,796	22,659	3.4
Boarding and retail costs	4,612	28,311	4.3
Total cost of professional services	14,736	164,862	25.0
GROSS PROFIT	45,677	495,646	75.0
OPERATING EXPENSES			
Doctor and staff costs			
Owner's compensation	12,500	150,000	22.7
Staff salaries and wages	14,011	169,090	25.6
Relief doctors	0	4,566	0.7
Payroll taxes	2,227	25,846	3.9
Health insurance	208	25,743	3.9
Retirement plan contributions	7,977	7,977	1.2
Continuing education	0	2,762	0.4
Total doctor and staff costs	36,923	385,984	58.4
Equipment costs			
Maintenance/service contracts	63	761	0.1
Depreciation on furniture and equipment	4,945	4,945	0.7
Amortization of computer software	1,678	1,678	0.3
Personal property taxes	0	581	0.1
Total equipment costs	6,686	7,965	1.2
Facility costs			
Rent on practice facility	3,050	38,970	5.9
Depreciation on leasehold improvements	784	784	0.1
Insurance on practice facility	0	890	0.1
Repairs on practice facility	83	613	0.1
Utilities	540	6,451	1.0
Total facility costs	4,457	47,708	7.2
General and administrative costs			
Accounting services	250	1,175	0.2
Advertising and promotion	275	698	0.1
Auto expenses/mileage reimbursements	177	2,647	0.4
Charitable contributions	50	250	0.0
Interest expense	176	2,031	0.3
Laundry and uniforms	130	681	0.1
Meals and entertainment	485	865	0.1
Office supplies	176	3,928	0.6
Postage	85	781	0.1
Printing	59	476	0.1
Professional liability insurance	0	3,300	0.5
Sales and use tax remitted	318	4,495	0.7
Telephone	412	4,997	0.8
Total general and administrative costs	2,593	26,324	4.0
Total operating expenses	50,659	467,981	70.9
INCOME FROM OPERATIONS	(4,982)	27,665	4.2
Other income (expense)	0	0	0.0
INCOME BEFORE TAXES	(4,982)	27,665	4.2
Less income tax	0	0	0.0
NET INCOME	($4,982)	$27,665	4.2

TABLE 7.2   Historical Balance Sheets

XYZ Animal Hospital, Inc.
Statement of Assets, Liabilities, and Equity-Income Tax Basis
December 31, 20X5

ASSETS		
Petty cash	$150	
Checking account	22,600	
Money market funds	34,950	
Accounts receivable	0	
Due from officer	1,000	
Drugs and supply inventory	19,820	
Total current assets		$78,520
Medical and surgical equipment	$250,680	
Less accumulated depreciation	(246,812)	
Office equipment, furniture, and fixtures	96,822	
Less accumulated depreciation	(87,900)	
Software	41,160	
Less accumulated amortization	(36,500)	
Leasehold improvements	126,750	
Less accumulated depreciation	(85,300)	
Net property and equipment		58,900
TOTAL ASSETS		$137,420
LIABILITIES		
Accounts payable	$0	
Line of credit	9,800	
Payroll taxes payable	2,415	
Accrued retirement plan payable	6,870	
Total current liabilities		$19,085
Long-term debt		24,050
TOTAL LIABILITIES		$43,135
SHAREHOLDER'S EQUITY		
Common stock		$1,500
Retained earnings		92,785
TOTAL SHAREHOLDER'S EQUITY		$94,285
TOTAL LIABILITIES AND EQUITY		$137,420

First, the valuator determines that Dr. Smith's outstanding receivables due from clients increased during the year by $3,873. In other words, his accounts receivable at the end of 20x5 were that much higher than the receivables at the beginning of the year. To adjust the figures to an accrual basis instead of a cash basis, the revenue (called "fees for services" in the tables) for the year should be increased by the same amount. Therefore, as adjustment (1), Dr. Smith's fees for services ($596,297) are increased by $3,873, and the adjusted gross revenue becomes $600,170 (see "Adjustments" column of Table 7.3).

Second, the appraiser needs to adjust the number entered for Dr. Smith's compensation. Dr. Smith was actually paid $150,000 for his services during 20x5. However, for the purposes of the appraisal, the amount of the owner's compensation must be based on industry statistics, not the actual amount of the owner's salary. The appraiser must determine what it would cost to replace Dr. Smith, both as a veterinarian and as a manager, at current rates for the area. Using his reference materials, he finds that for this locale and for the amount of business the owner generates, the appropriate compensation for veterinary services would be $109,200, or $40,800 less than Dr. Smith was paid. That amount is shown as adjustment (2) in Table 7.3. In addition, the appraiser believes Dr. Smith is entitled to an additional 2% of adjusted gross revenue (that is, 2% of $600,170), or $12,003, for his services in overseeing the practice operations, which becomes adjustment (3). Therefore, Dr. Smith's total adjusted compensation is $121,203, or $28,797 less than he was actually paid. This means that a portion of Dr. Smith's compensation actually represented practice profits.

The valuator also looks at staff compensation. Dr. Smith's spouse draws a salary from the practice in order to qualify for retirement benefits, and their daughter works during breaks from school. Based on their actual duties—and substituting current hourly rates for their work—the appraiser determines that their combined compensation is $24,000 higher than what a buyer would pay an unrelated person or persons to perform those services. This becomes adjustment (4). All other staff members are unrelated to Dr. Smith and their compensation was determined to be reasonable.

Payroll taxes would be lower if Dr. Smith was paid less and his wife and daughter were paid less. The appraiser calculates that the payroll taxes would in fact be $4,276 lower. This is shown as adjustment (5).

Similarly, the company has been making a contribution to both Dr. Smith's and Mrs. Smith's retirement plan accounts, as well as contributions to retirement plans

TABLE 7.3   Calculations of Adjusted Earnings

XYZ Animal Hospital, Inc.
Calculations of Adjusted Earnings
For the 12 Months Ended
December 31, 20X5

	Historical Income & Expenses	Adjustments		Adjusted Income & Expenses
INCOME FROM OPERATIONS				
Fees for services	$596,297	3,873	(1)	$600,170
Boarding and retail	64,211			64,211
Total income from operations	660,508			664,381
COST OF PROFESSIONAL SERVICES				
Drugs and medical supplies	93,022			93,022
Laboratory costs	20,870			20,870
Imaging costs	22,659			22,659
Boarding and retail costs	28,311			28,311
Total cost of professional services	164,862			164,862
GROSS PROFIT	495,646			499,519
OPERATING EXPENSES				
Doctor and staff costs				
Owner's compensation	150,000	(40,800)	(2)	109,200
Owner's management compensation	0	12,003	(3)	12,003
Staff salaries and wages	169,090	(24,000)	(4)	145,090
Relief doctors	4,566			4,566
Payroll taxes	25,846	(4,276)	(5)	21,570
Health insurance	25,743			25,743
Retirement plan contributions	7,977	(1,620)	(6)	6,357
Continuing education	2,762			2,762
Total doctor and staff costs	385,984			327,291
Equipment costs				
Maintenance/service contracts	761			761
Depreciation and amortization expense	6,623	(6,623)	(7)	0
Personal property taxes	581			581
Economic depreciation/replacement/repair	0	6,644	(8)	6,644
Total equipment costs	7,965			7,986
Facility costs				
Rent on practice facility	38,970			38,970
Depreciation on leasehold improvements	784	(784)	(9)	0
Insurance on practice facility	890			890
Repairs on practice facility	613			613
Utilities	6,451			6,451
Total facility costs	47,708			46,924
General and administrative costs				
Accounting services	1,175			1,175
Advertising and promotion	698			698
Auto expenses/mileage reimbursements	2,647	(950)	(10)	1,697
Charitable contributions	250	(250)	(11)	0
Interest expense	2,031	(2,031)	(12)	0
Laundry and uniforms	681			681
Meals and entertainment	865			865
Office supplies	3,928			3,928
Postage	781			781
Printing	476			476
Professional liability insurance	3,300			3,300
Sales and use tax remitted	4,495			4,495
Telephone	4,997			4,997
Total general and administrative costs	26,324			23,093
Total operating expenses	467,981			405,295
INCOME FROM OPERATIONS	27,665			94,224
Other income (expense)	0			0
INCOME BEFORE TAXES	27,665			94,225
Less income tax	0			0
NET INCOME	$27,665			$94,225

on behalf of the other eligible employees. The contribution for 20x5 was larger than it would have been if both Dr. and Mrs. Smith had been receiving the more modest wages described above. The excess contribution ($1,620) is added back in as a discretionary item. This is adjustment (6). Their daughter did not participate in the retirement plan, since she did not work enough hours to become eligible.

Next, the appraiser adds back depreciation on the practice's equipment and leasehold improvements as well as the amortization expense on the practice's computer software, since these are non-cash expenses. Then he subtracts an estimate of economic depreciation, or an estimate of wear and tear and annual equipment replacement necessary to keep the equipment up-to-date. These are shown as adjustments (7), (8), and (9).

The practice pays Dr. Smith's auto expenses and reimburses staff members for business mileage at the current IRS rate. Dr. Smith has informed the appraiser that approximately 52% of the expenses for his car is business-related, while the other 48% is not. Adding back 48% of his auto expenses results in adjustment (10), an addition of $950 to net income. No adjustment is made for the staff reimbursements, since those are business-related.

The valuator adds back the charitable contributions made during the year as adjustment (11), since these are discretionary.

Finally, the interest expense of $2,031 is added back as adjustment (12). Interest represents an expense related to a practice's capitalization (mix of debt versus equity) rather than an operating expense. Since Dr. Smith will be paying off this debt from the proceeds of the sale, this will not be a recurring expense for the buyer, even though the purchaser will likely be paying interest on new debt taken out to buy the practice.

These adjustments, taken together, mean that although the practice's historical net income was only $27,665, a more accurate figure for appraisal purposes would be $94,225. This figure is shown on the bottom line in Table 7.3. It represents the "adjusted earnings," or "income before taxes," for the practice. This practice is a pass-through entity, meaning that the owner pays income taxes personally on the practice profits, and the practice itself pays no income taxes. Most veterinary practice appraisals currently are prepared on a pretax basis, since the majority of practices operate as pass-through entities and the owners' personal tax rates vary widely because of factors independent of the practices themselves.

The adjustments described above are based on the purpose and standard of value determined for this valuation. Using the same basic facts, the adjustments would be different, and adjusted earnings would be different, if the appraiser was valuing the practice for an associate buy-in. In that case, the buyer would be purchasing an undivided piece of the practice's equity, not 100% of its assets. And since associates generally buy a noncontrolling interest, some of the adjustments described above might not represent reality after the buy-in. For example, if another owner was buying into the practice, but Dr. Smith was still going to pay his spouse and daughter the additional $24,000 in annual compensation, then those dollars would not be available for profit distributions after the buy-in, and no adjustment would be made. It is critical that the adjustments made to arrive at the adjusted earnings figure represent what is really likely to occur. Otherwise, the associate may well be paying an unrealistic price for his or her share of the practice.

Calculating the Value of Practice Assets

Once the adjustments are made, the appraiser may begin step 7, calculating the value of the assets or equity in the practice, depending on the purpose of the valuation and the facts of the case. We'll use the same facts to demonstrate three different income approaches to valuation: the single-period capitalization method, the excess earnings method, and the discounted cash flow (or discounted earnings) method. These are the most commonly used methods, and, if done properly, each can result in a reasonable (and similar) conclusion of value.

Applying the Single-Period Capitalization Method

Table 7.4 reflects the valuator's calculation of the value of the practice assets, including goodwill, using the single-period capitalization method.

The underlying theory behind this approach is that the practice's adjusted earnings are the result of the actual pool of assets within the practice, a pool that will vary from one practice to another. Those assets include equipment, inventory, use of the facility, doctors and staff, goodwill, and so on. In other words, this method makes no distinction between tangible and intangible assets and makes no attempt to value them separately. It assumes a single rate of return for all assets, rather than different rates of return for tangible and intangible assets. The only assets that are not included in the pool are those that will not be sold as part of the hypothetical sale, and they are detailed below.

The selling price of the assets does not necessarily reflect everything the seller will receive at closing. There may be other assets (primarily cash) that the seller will retain outside of the sale, and the seller may also be responsible for paying off the practice's debts. (The buyer may, however, specifically agree to assume a particular debt, such as an equipment lease.)

Table 7.4 starts with adjusted earnings from each of the previous five years. The valuator would have made adjustments as needed for years 20x1 through 20x4 just as she did for year 20x5. The resulting adjusted earnings figures are shown in the top row of the table. Next, the valuator calculates average adjusted earnings in two different ways. First, by giving the greatest weight to the most recent year, the valuator calculates average adjusted earnings under an assumption that 20x5 is a better approximation of future earnings than any of the four previous years. The weighting formula used must be based on the facts of a given practice; there are many different formulas that can be used. The choice should be explained in the report. In this case, average weighted adjusted earnings turn out to be $78,210. The second calculation is a simple average, giving equal weight to all the years, and results in average adjusted earnings of $71,831.

TABLE 7.4   Single–Period Capitalization Method

XYZ Animal Hospital, Inc.
Calculation of the Value of the Assets Using
CAPITALIZED EARNINGS METHOD
as of December 31, 20X5

	20X5	**20X4**	**20X3**	**20X2**	**20X1**
Adjusted earnings	$94,224	$81,466	$62,875	$66,940	$53,652
Weighting	5	4	3	2	1
Weighted earnings	471,122	325,864	188,625	133,880	53,652
Total weighted earnings	1,173,143				
Divided by sum of weights	15				
Average weighted adjusted earnings	78,210				
Adjusted earnings	$94,224	$81,466	$62,875	$66,940	$53,652
Equal weighting	1	1	1	1	1
Weighted earnings	94,224	81,466	62,875	66,940	53,652
Total weighted earnings	359,157				
Divided by sum of weights	5				
Average adjusted earnings	71,831				

Average weighted adjusted earnings in the next year (one year's growth)	80,947
Capitalization rate[1]	19.7%
Value of the practice assets	$410,898
Rounded	$415,000

1. Capitalization rate was determined using an analysis of the Ibbotson/Morningstar buildup method and Duff & Phelps 25th portfolio using total assets, sales, and five-year EBITDA. Go to http://corporate.morningstar.com/ib/asp/subject.aspx?xmlfile=1422.xml and www. bvresources.com for more information.

In calculating the value of the assets, the valuator decides to use the weighted average, or $78,210. This figure will be divided by the capitalization rate to determine the value of the practice's assets. However, that figure is increased by one year's estimated growth, since it represents earnings in the next year, not earnings in the year that ended on the valuation date.

The capitalization rate, 19.7% in this case, is shown near the bottom of the table. Depending on the method the valuator used to determine the capitalization rate, the underlying math may not be disclosed in the report. However, there should be an explanation of how the rate was determined, the factors the appraiser considered, and how he views this practice's risk as compared with other veterinary practices. Above all, the appraiser should not pull a number out of the air and expect you to believe it represents any practice's expected rate of return. In Dr. Smith's situation, a capitalization rate of 19.7% suggests a practice with a steady earnings stream. It also reflects the risk inherent in the profession overall and in this particular practice. For example, a limited pool of buyers is available in a private market, particularly when it comes to veterinary practices. Also, for Dr. Smith's practice, the facility rent may increase at the time of the lease renewal, or the practice may outgrow the facility and be forced to relocate. The capitalization rate the appraiser chooses must take all of this into consideration, which is why determining the capitalization rate takes skill and experience.

One of the potential traps of using the single-period capitalization method is that the pool of assets may include nonoperating assets that are not identified during the appraisal process. If, for example, a practice is accumulating cash toward the purchase of a new facility by investing in marketable securities, those investments are not operating assets. If the practice value is simply based on capitalizing adjusted earnings, then the implication is that the extra cash is needed for operations and is part of the sale.

The same would be true for equipment that is owned or leased by the practice, but not being efficiently used. If a practice buys ultrasound equipment but has no one trained to use it, then the equipment becomes a nonoperating asset. In these situations, the valuator must determine whether each of the assets is actually being used as part of the operations and helps to generate profits. If not, that asset must be pulled out of the pool before the adjusted earnings are capitalized to determine the value of the practice. The seller may choose to retain nonoperating assets (like the marketable securities) and disclose to the buyer that they are not part of the sale. Alternatively, if the buyer wants the nonoperating assets (like the ultrasound equipment), they can be added to the value of the practice to arrive at the price a buyer should pay for the entire bundle of assets.

Table 7.4 reflects the valuator's conclusion that the practice's assets are worth $415,000 (rounded). The appraiser's mathematics resulted in a figure of $410,898, but practice values are actually not that precise. Some valuators state their conclusion in the form of a range ($410,000 to $420,000, for example), while others simply round the result, as in this case. Note that the seller would also keep the practice's cash, or an additional $57,700, as of the date of the valuation, since buyers rarely buy cash.

Applying the Excess Earnings Method

The second method is based on the assumption that there is a different rate of return expected from tangible versus intangible assets because the risk of creating profits from each of those categories is different. For many years, this was the method of choice for veterinary practice appraisers, and it is still fairly commonly used. (See Table 7.5.)

Even though this calculation starts with adjusted earnings, some appraisers believe that it is an asset method as well as an income method. In any case, it presumes that with intangibles, there is both greater risk and greater return than with tangibles. The method therefore breaks adjusted earnings into two pieces: a return on net tangible assets and a return on intangible assets. To do this, the valuator calculates adjusted earnings as described in the previous method and then subtracts the expected return on tangible assets. If he determines that the rate on tangibles is 8.4%, then the value of the inventory, equipment, furniture, leasehold improvements, and other tangible assets is summed up; reduced by the liabilities related directly to those assets, if any; and then multiplied by 8.4%, as shown in Table 7.5.

The difference between average weighted adjusted earnings and the calculated return on tangible assets represents the return on the intangibles. The valuator then divides the portion of the earnings related to the intangibles by a capitalization rate determined just for the intangibles. The value of the tangible assets is then added to the calculated value of the intangibles to arrive at the total value of the practice assets.

TABLE 7.5   Excess Earnings Method

XYZ Animal Hospital, Inc.
Calculation of the Value of the Assets Using the
EXCESS EARNINGS METHOD
as of December 31, 20X5

	20X5		**20X4**	**20X3**	**20X2**	**20X1**
Adjusted earnings	$94,224		$81,466	$62,875	$66,940	$53,652
Weighting	5		4	3	2	1
Weighted earnings	471,122		325,864	188,625	133,880	53,652
Total weighted earnings	1,173,143					
Divided by sum of weights	15					
Average weighted adjusted earnings	78,210					
Adjusted earnings	$94,224		$81,466	$62,875	$66,940	$53,652
Equal weighting	1		1	ˋ1	1	1
Weighted earnings	94,224		81,466	62,875	66,940	53,652
Total weighted earnings	359,157					
Divided by sum of weights	5					
Average adjusted earnings	71,831					

Average weighted adjusted earnings	78,210	
Value of the net tangible assets		251,765
× Return on tangible assets[1]		8.4%
− Earnings attributed to tangibles	(21,148)	
= Earnings attributed to intangibles	57,061	
÷ Cap rate for intangibles[2]	35.2%	
= Value of the intangibles		162,105
Value of the net tangible practice assets	$251,765	
Value of the intangible assets	162,105	
Total value	$413,870	
Rounded	$415,000	

1. Capitalization rate was determined from an analysis of the owner's cost of capital based on current rates on his debt and his estimated rate on shareholder's equity.
2. Capitalization rate was determined using an analysis of the Ibbotson/Morningstar buildup method and Duff & Phelps 25th portfolio using total assets, sales, and five-year EBITDA. For more information, go to http://corporate.morningstar.com/ib/asp/subject.aspx?xmlfile=1422.xml and www.bvresources.com.

Table 7.5 shows the calculation based on the facts in our case study. Note particularly that the capitalization rate used in calculating the goodwill value is different from the capitalization rate shown in Table 7.4 for the single-period capitalization method. That's because the capitalization rate in Table 7.5 was determined solely for the intangible assets, which carry a higher risk. Because the risk is higher, the capitalization rate must be higher. (Higher cap rates generate lower values, while lower cap rates result in higher values. For example, $100,000 of earnings capitalized at 7% generates over $1.4 million in value [$100,000 divided by 0.07], whereas the same $100,000 capitalized at 20% suggests a $500,000 value [$100,000 divided by 0.20].)

Although the excess earnings method has commonly been used in the veterinary profession, it is losing ground. To a large extent that is because it is easy to misuse the method. There are four main reasons for this:

- First, the value of the tangible assets is frequently only an estimate, because the equipment, furniture, and software were not actually appraised to determine their fair market value. Let's say that Dr. Smith and the valuator agreed to use a list of the assets, their acquisition dates, and their original cost as the basis for estimating their fair market value as of December 31, 20x5. If the estimate they produce is higher than their actual value, then the portion of the adjusted earnings attributed to the tangible assets will be artificially high and the return on the intangibles will be artificially low. The result will be that goodwill is undervalued.

- Second, most valuators estimate the return on tangible assets without looking at the practice's actual cost of capital. In other words, what rate would that particular practice have to pay to finance those tangible assets? Most loans require at least a down payment by the owner, but what is the return on equity that would entice the owner to invest his or her own money (as equity) rather than borrowing it? Not surprisingly, practices with higher debt loads must pay more to borrow money, and at some point cannot borrow at all. Therefore, the expected return on tangible assets should vary from practice to practice, though in reality we see only a narrow range of percentages used for the return on tangible assets.

- Third, the number or range of values arrived at for a practice should be fairly similar regardless of the valuation method used, assuming the same purpose, standard of value, and valuation date, but with this method practices with more tangible assets would be expected to have lower goodwill value. That's because more of the adjusted earnings would be attributable to tangible assets, not the excess earnings used to calculate the value of the goodwill. But it doesn't seem logical that practices with fewer tangible assets would have higher goodwill value simply because the return on tangible assets is a smaller portion of the total adjusted earnings.

- Finally, to keep the values the same between methods, those practices with more tangible assets would need to have a higher capitalization rate on the intangible assets to keep the overall values comparable. But does having more equipment, for example, cause a practice to be riskier than one with less invested in tangible assets?

Overall, the valuator determined that the value of Dr. Smith's practice assets was still $415,000 by using the excess earnings method. The actual math produced a slightly higher number ($413,870 versus $410,898) than was calculated in Table 7.4, but the difference is less than 1% of the practice's value.

Applying the Discounted Cash Flow (or Discounted Earnings) Method

Our third method takes a very different approach to valuation because it is based on forecasted earnings, not historical results. This method is based on the belief that a buyer of a practice is actually buying the stream of profits (or cash flow) that the practice can generate in the future, restated in today's dollars.

The buyer is assumed to ask the question, "How long will it take to get my money back if I expect an annual return of X percent, given what I think will happen over the next few years?" Rather than looking at historical earnings, the valuator will use forecasted earnings as the basis of the calculation. Outside the veterinary profession, and among investors who buy other kinds of businesses, this is the preferred income method. These investors are less interested in the past results of operations than in future earnings.

Although this method is used less frequently than other methods in veterinary practice valuations, it is likely the preferred method when the practice's expected profits in the future will not represent a steady earnings stream when compared with the past. If, for example, a referral practice is adding a new specialty and a new specialist, past earnings will not be a good representation of what will happen in the future. Similarly, a practice going through an extensive remodel of its current facility or moving into a new one will likely have the capacity to produce more revenue, though there are costs involved in the facility expansion itself and in the employees who will generate that new revenue.

Logistically, this method has some difficulties. Few practice owners are adept at budgeting income and expenses, and most in fact have little or no experience with creating budgets and monitoring actual results. Therefore, the owners of the practice being valued are probably not proficient in developing forecasted earnings. Those who have used budgets for several years may have improved their projection skills from year to year and are more likely to produce accurate predictions; with those who have not used budgets, the accuracy of the projections is anybody's guess. A valuator cannot simply ask for projections and assume they represent realistic expectations. Unfortunately, veterinary practice owners generally are not experienced business planners.

As a result, when future operations are likely to be very different from past operations because of a major change in the facility, the services offered, or staffing, the valuator may ask the practice owners to work with their Certified Public Accountant to develop these forecasts. Among other things, the practice owner will need help analyzing the costs involved in generating additional revenue. The valuator can then review the projections and underlying assumptions for reasonableness without being involved in the development of the projected figures themselves. Many valuators believe that developing the projections creates a potential conflict of interest for an appraiser—hence the need for the involvement of an experienced CPA.

Table 7.6 reflects some modifications in the facts of our case study in order to make discounted future earnings an appropriate method for this practice. The actual calculation of the value is then reflected on that schedule. Although the calculation looks complex, the concepts are fairly simple. The adjusted figure for net income in 20x5 from Table 7.3 is shown at the top of the far left column. Just as in the previous methods, actual depreciation and amortization are added back but no economic depreciation is subtracted. Similarly, non-cash expenditures and interest expense are also added back. Additional assumptions are also provided that reflect the capital expenditures (for equipment, for example) the practice made in that year and the working capital (current assets less current liabilities) it needed to fund those expenditures. The result is net cash flow for 20x5.

Net income for each of the next five years is also projected, along with capital expenditures and working capital needs. As shown in the table, the practice is projecting significant growth in net income over the period of the projections as a result of investing in new equipment, hiring additional staff, and growing the practice overall. However, the owner predicts that the growth will then level off. Normalized earnings are shown in the far right column.

Using standard present value tables or a financial calculator, the appraiser uses a present value factor of 26.8% for each of the five years, designed to reflect the time value of money. Logically, one would expect the current value of profit to be earned in the fifth year to be a smaller percentage of actual profit than the profit to be earned next year. The 20x6 factor is therefore 78.86%, while the factor in the fifth year is 30.51.%.

Finally, businesses don't last forever, and so the valuator must estimate a terminal value to reflect that the earnings stream won't go on indefinitely. In this case, the present value of the terminal net cash flow (estimated at $180,000) is capitalized using the assumptions shown and then discounted back to present dollars using the present value factor for the fifth year. The resulting figure, the present value of terminal net cash flow, represents the future profits in the sixth and future years,

TABLE 7.6   Discounted Cash Flow Method

XYZ Animal Hospital, Inc.
Calculation of the Value of the Assets Using
DISCOUNTED CASH FLOW METHOD
as of December 31, 20X5

Assumptions

Historical facts are the same as in the original case study, except for these modifications:
Dr. Smith plans to undertake a $120,000 remodel to expand the usable space in the facility.
Dr. Smith plans to borrow $100,000 at 7% interest to pay for the remodel.
Dr. Smith has estimated the new equipment and additional cash he will need each year.

Present Value of Projected Cash Flows

	20X5 Adjusted Cash Flow	20X6 Projected	20X7 Projected	20X8 Projected	20X9 Projected	20X0 Projected	Norm. 20X0
Net income	$94,224	$108,648	$146,777	$185,300	$211,543	$215,420	$215,420
Plus depreciation and amortization	6,644	20,255	6,861	7,952	12,268	8,806	–
Plus interest expense, net of taxes	0	5,250	3,675	2,888	2,048	1,260	1,260
Less capital expenditures	(1,620)	(120,000)	(15,000)	(15,000)	(22,500)	(9,500)	–
Less working capital requirements¹	(2,635)	60,000	(43,100)	(39,000)	(37,850)	(35,300)	(35,300)
Net cash flow	96,613	74,153	99,213	142,140	165,509	180,686	181,380
× Present value factor (@ 26.8%)		0.78864	0.62196	0.4905	0.38683	0.30507	
= Present value of projected cash flows		$58,480	$61,707	$69,719	$64,024	$55,122	

Total present value of interim cash flows $309,051

1. 20X6 = $100,000 loan proceeds less $40,000 additional working capital.

Present Value of Terminal Net Cash Flow

20X1 net cash flow	$180,000
Capitalization rate (midyear cash flows, 4% growth)	22.8%
Terminal value (net cash flow divided by capitalization rate)	789,474
x Present value factor at 26.8%	0.305
= Present value of terminal cash flow	$240,845

Valuation Summary

Value of interim cash flows	$309,051
Value of terminal cash flows	240,845
Value of invested capital	$549,895
Rounded	$550,000

restated as a present value. The practice value is the sum of the present value of the projected cash flow for the next five years plus the value of the terminal (sixth year forward) cash flows. This sum represents invested capital, some of which would come from debt and some of which would come from the owner (equity).

The value of the practice in this example is just under $550,000, somewhat higher than when using the first two methods. However, the difference is due to the change in facts, not the method itself. In other words, we were predicting only a moderate annual growth in earnings under the first two methods. But when using discounted cash flow, we changed the facts about the practice and assumed that it was expected to experience significant growth over the next few years and would be borrowing money to fund that expansion. It is those new factors that create the increase in value, not the choice of valuation method.

Some errors that are common with the discounted cash flow method. One can occur when matching the discount rate to the benefit stream. When using this method, the valuator must decide which benefit stream is to be discounted, as there are several options. The choice could be discounted cash flow to equity, discounted cash flow to invested capital (debt and equity), or discounted earnings, among others. While a discussion of these options and the concepts behind them is beyond the scope of this publication, it is important to understand that anyone using this method should have a thorough understanding of how to use it properly.

A second problem is that although projecting increased revenue is fairly easy, predicting the increase in expenses and necessary capital to fund that growth is much more difficult. Yet logic tells us that it takes cash to grow a business, and that cash must come from the owners, from the practice's earnings, or from debt. Overlooking some of the necessary expenditures can lead to a rosy picture of the future that is unsupported by the true facts.

Another issue is a tendency to overlook the terminal value. No earnings stream can be expected to go on forever, and the terminal value is designed to acknowledge that there will be an end. In addition, with each future year, the value of the earnings in that year is lower in today's dollars, so at some point the current value of the profit in some future year is essentially zero. The higher the present value factor, the sooner that happens.

Finally, this method is especially vulnerable to even small changes in the various inputs. To demonstrate this, it is often helpful for the valuator to create a sensitivity table illustrating the impact on the practice value when the discount rate, terminal value, growth rate, and future earnings are modified.

Adjusting the Balance Sheet

Regardless of the method chosen to come up with a practice value, buyers and sellers must allocate the value among the assets. Both buyer and seller must use the same allocations, and they each must disclose these allocations when their tax returns are prepared for the year of the transaction. For that reason, many valuators include an adjusted balance sheet setting forth suggested prices for groups of assets and reflecting any liabilities that are part of the transaction.

The assets, including goodwill, as well as the liabilities are all restated to their current values, which can be either higher or lower than their cost on the historical financial statements. Table 7.7 is an example of an adjusted balance sheet determined under the single-period capitalization method. Here, several adjustments were made to reflect an estimate of the current value of the practice's assets, including goodwill.

The adjustments labeled as (1) account for the fact that this is a fair market value appraisal and we expect the buyer to purchase the practice assets, not its equity. In other words, buyers do not purchase the practice's cash, so the cash balances are removed from the adjusted balance sheet. However, it is important to note that this cash will be retained by the seller and will be available to pay off the practice's liabilities.

Even though the practice's historical balance sheet at the end of 20x5 shows no accounts receivable because it was prepared using the cash method of accounting, there were in fact outstanding accounts due from clients in the amount of $33,844 at the end of the year, according to the practice management software. The appraiser determined that the value of these, based on age and collectibility, is $21,945, and added that figure as adjustment (2). It is generally preferable that the buyer purchase the outstanding accounts at a discounted price reflecting the likelihood of collecting these accounts, since otherwise clients with outstanding accounts would receive confusing invoices with two different payees for before and after the sale of the practice.

"Due from officer" in the asset section refers to a loan Dr. Smith made to himself from the practice two years ago in December when he needed cash for the holidays. Because he didn't want to increase his personal tax liability, he took it as a loan instead of a bonus. He had always intended to repay the money, but he probably won't do that if he sells the practice. Therefore, it is removed as adjustment (3).

The drug and supply inventory was physically counted and priced as of December 31, 20x5. The cost of the inventory at that time was $19,820, and only a minor adjustment was needed to adjust the practice management software figure at that date to the actual physical count. The appraiser is comfortable using that figure, and Dr. Smith has indicated that there have been no material changes in quantities or prices since then.

Dr. Smith and the valuator agreed in their preliminary discussions that he would not hire a personal property appraiser to value his furniture and equipment. The valuator told him that this would be disclosed in his report as a limiting factor, and Dr. Smith agreed to provide him with an accurate list of the individual items now in use in the practice, their original cost, and their current condition. Together they developed current values for the equipment, furniture, and software.

Dr. Smith's list includes a few items acquired several years ago that were written off the books when they were fully depreciated but are still in use, including a microscope and two small file cabinets. In addition, he understands that the leasehold improvements (tenant finish) have limited value to a buyer since they revert to the landlord at the end of the lease. However, he believes that a buyer would continue to occupy the current facility for several years. The valuator agreed to put a $20,000 value on these leasehold improvements, even though their original cost

TABLE 7.7   Adjusted Balance Sheet

XYZ Animal Hospital, Inc.
Adjusted Assets, Liabilities and Equity
December 31, 20X5

ASSETS	Historical Balances	Adjustment		Adjusted Balances	
Petty cash	$150	(150)	(1)	$0	
Checking account	22,600	(22,600)	(1)	0	
Money market funds	34,950	(34,950)	(1)	0	
Accounts receivable (net)	0	21,945	(2)	21,945	
Due from officer	1,000	(1,000)	(3)	0	
Drugs and supply inventory	19,820			19,820	
Total current assets	78,520			41,765	
Medical and surgical equipment	250,680	(115,680)	(4)	135,000	
Less accumulated depreciation	(246,812)	246,812	(4)	0	
Office equipment, furniture, and fixtures	96,822	(61,822)	(5)	35,000	
Less accumulated depreciation	(87,900)	87,900	(5)	0	
Software	41,160	(21,160)	(6)	20,000	
Less accumulated amortization	(36,500)	36,500	(6)	0	
Leasehold improvements	126,750	(106,750)	(7)	20,000	
Less accumulated depreciation	(85,300)	85,300	(7)	0	
Net property and equipment	58,900			210,000	
Goodwill	0	163,235	(8)	163,235	
TOTAL ASSETS	$137,420			**$415,000**	Asset Value
LIABILITIES					
Accounts payable	0			0	
Line of credit	9,800	(9,800)	(9)	0	
Payroll taxes payable	2,415	(2,415)	(9)	0	
Accrued retirement plan payable	6,870	(6,870)	(9)	0	
Total current liabilities	19,085			0	
Long-term debt	24,050	(24,050)	(9)	0	
TOTAL LIABILITIES	43,135			0	
SHAREHOLDER'S EQUITY	94,285	320,715	(10)	415,000	
TOTAL LIABILITIES AND EQUITY	$137,420			$415,000	

was over $126,000. The adjustments to add the microscope and file cabinets, to substitute estimated current value for cost, and to add back all accumulated depreciation and amortization are shown as adjustments (4) through (7).

Adjustment (8) records the value of the goodwill, calculated on this schedule as the difference between the value of the total assets being sold and the total adjusted value of the tangible assets.

The outstanding debt of the practice at the end of the year was based on a review of payments made to vendors in January 20x6 and other information given to the appraiser. He has computed accounts payable at $16,500, which is approximately the amount at the end of 20x5. The appraiser made no adjustment for this item, as the buyer will expect Dr. Smith to pay off the practice debts from the sale proceeds by using the practice's cash on hand and in the bank.

The lease for the clinic's space is not recorded as a liability; instead, rent payments are expensed to the income statement as the checks are written. All payments have been made on time, and the current lease will expire in four years. The primary term of the lease was five years. However, several renewal options are built into the lease that call for rent at the market rate at that time. It has been determined that the lease is at fair market value based on the current market conditions in Dr. Smith's locale. The lease is transferable with the permission of the landlord, which is why the valuator believes the buyer will be willing to pay for a portion of the original tenant finish, as discussed for Adjustment (7).

Since this lease was determined to be at fair market value, and the practice must operate somewhere, the total payments are not recorded as a liability on the balance sheet. If the obligation had been determined to be higher than lease terms on comparable space now, the difference between the actual lease payments due and the market lease rate would be added as a liability. If the reverse was true and the lease terms were more favorable to the clinic than a current lease, the difference would be added as an asset to the balance sheet.

The appraiser has reviewed Dr. Smith's retirement plan documents and determined that the company contribution for the year is properly reflected as a liability as of December 31. All employee contributions were deposited to their accounts by the due dates.

The terms of the long-term debt appear reasonable, and payments are being made as scheduled. Again, the seller will be responsible for paying off this debt. To reflect this fact, all of the practice liabilities were adjusted to zero as adjustment (9).

The most significant adjustment is to the shareholder's equity section. Equity is a calculated number that when added to total liabilities *must* equal assets. The shareholder's equity figure in the far right column becomes the adjusted net book value of the assets and will be used in the practice value summary in the report. Adjustment (10) records this equity.

Prepare the Report

Early in the discussions with the valuator, the appraiser and Dr. Smith discussed what the valuation report would look like and what it would include. The engagement letter he signed indicated the type of report to be produced. Based on that agreement, the valuator prepares a report that meets Dr. Smith's objectives and adequately explains the results of the valuation process. The report also provides basic information about the practice, giving the potential buyer a better understanding of the practice, its services, its current ownership, and its unique characteristics.

Since these reports can be quite lengthy and can follow different formats, no sample report is included with this publication.

You should now have a better understanding of the valuation process for a veterinary practice. While appraisers wish that all valuations were as straightforward as this example, that is almost never the case. Similarly, valuators always hope for accurate, complete, and consistent practice data to work with. In reality, this does not happen very often either.

Understanding the valuation process can help you in both the short and the long term. If you are a buyer, keep in mind that good financial data benefit not just an appraiser but also the practice owner over the life of the practice. Recording expenses consistently and accurately provides better management information, as the practice owner can see how the data change over time and monitor trends accurately.

Knowing whether or not your practice is increasing in value helps you avoid ugly surprises when it's time for you to sell. A current owner may feel his or her practice is very profitable and therefore very valuable, but those same profits, from an appraiser's perspective, can be less impressive. When you understand how critical compensation, facility costs, drugs and supplies, and other major costs are to practice value, you can manage them more efficiently in a practice you own or one you plan to start or buy in the future.

About the Author

Lorraine Monheiser List, CPA, CVA, is a nationally recognized speaker, author, and consultant on financial and practice management issues for veterinarians and their teams. She works with wellness and specialty referral practices across the United States and in Canada. Lorraine graduated with honors from Colorado State University in accounting, earned her Certified Public Accountant designation, and then worked as a CPA specializing in tax for more than 20 years. After selling her accounting practice, she earned a master's degree in human resource development and cofounded Summit Veterinary Advisors to provide more in-depth services to the veterinary profession.

Lorraine holds a Certificate in Veterinary Practice Administration from the AAHA Veterinary Management Institute at Purdue University. After completing advanced valuation coursework, passing a comprehensive examination, and submitting a valuation report for review, Lorraine was granted the Certified Valuation Analyst designation by the National Association of Certified Valuation Analysts (NACVA). Lorraine, a charter member of VetPartners, recently served on its board of directors and as treasurer. She also cochairs the VetPartners Veterinary Valuation Resource Council.

Lorraine lives in the Denver metro area with her husband and the cat that owns them, and she has two sons, a stepson, a stepdaughter, and five grandsons.